Talk to Your Doc

The Patient's Guide

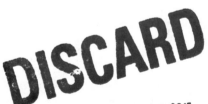

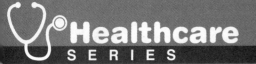

Healthcare
SERIES

Talk to Your Doc
The Patient's Guide

Mary F. Hawkins

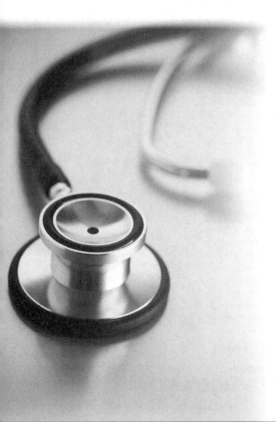

Self-Counsel Press
(a division of)
International Self-Counsel Press Ltd.
USA   Canada

Self-Counsel Press acknowledges the financial support of the Government of Canada through the Canada Book Fund for our publishing activities.

Printed in Canada.

First edition: 2015

Library and Archives Canada Cataloguing in Publication

Hawkins, Mary F., author
    Talk to your doc : the patient's guide / Mary F. Hawkins.

(Healthcare series)
Issued in print and electronic formats.
ISBN 978-1-77040-227-0 (pbk.).—ISBN 978-1-77040-978-1 (epub).—
ISBN 978-1-77040-979-8 (kindle)

Back cover photo taken by Jean-Marc Carisse, used with permission.

Self-Counsel Press
(a division of)
International Self-Counsel Press Ltd.

Bellingham, WA   North Vancouver, BC
        USA   Canada

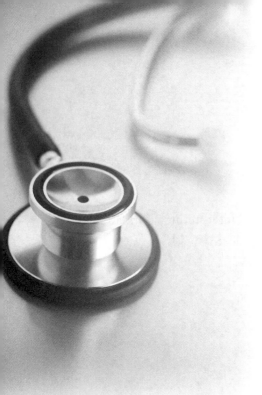

Contents

4 Communicating with Your Doctor

Checklists

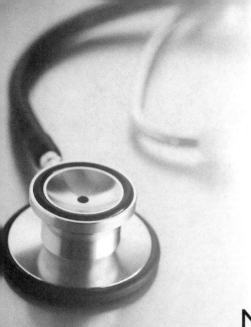

Notice to Readers

Laws are constantly changing. Every effort is made to keep this publication as current as possible. However, the author, the publisher, and the vendor of this book make no representations or warranties regarding the outcome or the use to which the information in this book is put and are not assuming any liability for any claims, losses, or damages arising out of the use of this book. The reader should not rely on the author or the publisher of this book for any professional advice. Please be sure that you have the most recent edition.

Website links often expire or web pages move, at the time of this book's publication the links were current.

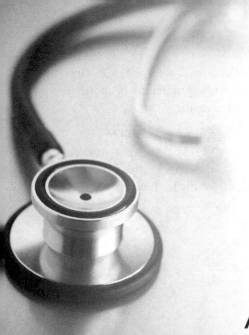

Acknowledgments

Special thanks to Nedra Lander, PhD; and the late Doris R. Hawkins; Dr. John E. Dawson, GP; and Andrea Lloyd, for their valued editorial comments and proofreading skills. Thank you to all the health-care professionals and patients who allowed me to interview them for the purpose of this book. A big thanks to others who voluntarily offered their expertise in proofreading skills and insights. All provided invaluable experience and suggestions that kept this book grounded in reality.

Thank you to Dr. Jeffrey Turnbull, Chief of Staff, Ottawa Hospital; Dr. David Hawkins, Executive Director Association of Canadian Medical Colleges; Dr. Paul Claman, Director of IVF-ET Program, and Associate Professor, University of Ottawa; Dr. John E. Dawson, GP; and Sharon Ann Kearns, BScN, CPHQ, Director of Quality/Performance and Risk at the University of Ottawa, Ottawa Hospital, Civic Site; and Cathy Beach, Specialist, Patient Advocacy Obstetrics, Gynecology, Newborn Care in the Ottawa Hospital. Their interviews and insights into patient-doctor relations helped me tremendously. Most of all, thank you to the individuals who participated in the focus groups on patient communication and who sent emails about their experiences.

Thank you, too, to the editors of the Canadian Medical Association Journal for publishing my request to interview physicians on patient communication in the magazine and on its website.

Thank you to my editor, Tanya Lee Howe, for her excellent editorial guidance. To all of those at Self-Counsel Press who have worked so hard to bring this book revision together. A special thank you to Kirk LaPointe, Publisher and Editor-in-Chief, for his faith in me, and for bringing this book to the North American market.

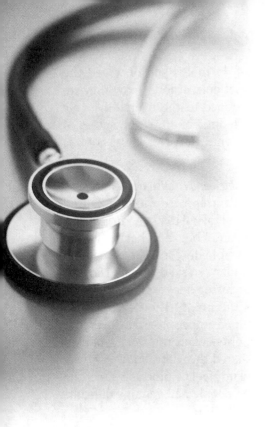

Preface

When I began teaching communication to university and college students, I often heard them say at the beginning of the course, "Communication, oh, that's easy. I'll get an A in this class." As the semester progressed they became perplexed and sometimes confused by the complexity of the communication process.

By the end of the term, many students told me how much they had learned from the lectures, group work, and discussions. They proudly told me how they now used what they had learned about communication in their everyday relationships. Many of these students matured through this process of learning.

My years of teaching oral and written communications, and personal interest led me to explore varied facets of communication, especially in the area of health. My graduate thesis was titled "Communicative Patterns and Leader Behaviour of Multi-Disciplinary Health Care Teams in Association with Team Cohesion and Team Culture." This study involved spending eight months with health-care teams in a central New York metropolitan hospital. I joined these teams three mornings a week at 5 a.m. I observed the interactions of surgeons and health-care professionals inside and outside of the operating rooms.

I also entered patient rooms with team members and observed the interactions between the doctors and patients. I noted how they responded to one another, and its importance to the overall dynamic of health care. It was this dynamic that led me to study the nature of communication between doctors and patients. However, it was not this alone that pulled me toward this topic.

In 1997, I wrote a book entitled *Unshielded: The Human Cost of the Dalkon Shield*. (The Dalkon Shield was a contraceptive device that caused women gynecological injury in the 1970s). I talked to many survivors of injury when I was researching the book, and I began to hear devastating complaints about negative responses from doctors. The perception of their experiences haunted these women. I asked them: "Did you ever tell the doctor how you felt about his or her response to you?" The reply was usually: "No, what was the point? The doctor would not listen anyway." My ear became attuned to people in my everyday encounters who described similar experiences in the doctor-patient relationship. Certainly, not all people shared this view, but there were enough that I wondered why people did not feel comfortable asserting themselves more. I concluded that some people had genuine difficulty in communicating their feelings to their doctors.

In the course of writing a weekly newspaper column on doctor-patient relations, I found confirmation of the latter conclusion in the complaints and questions I received from readers. I also conducted focus groups with patients as well as developed and gathered additional information via surveys. By now, I was well on my way to gathering anecdotes from these people I invited to the focus groups. They, among others, taught me that people voice their complaints to anyone who will listen — except to their doctor.

With the encouragement of many people, I have written *Talk to Your Doc*. It is my hope that this book will help you express how you feel to your doctor leading you to better health care.

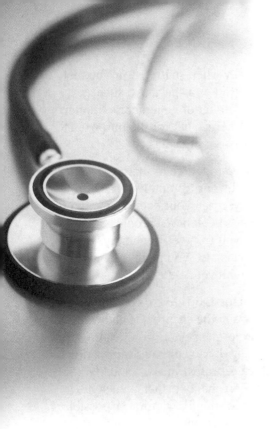

Introduction

At one time or another, most of us have complained to someone else about feeling dissatisfied with a visit with a doctor. Much of this dissatisfaction points to long waiting times, a doctor's rushed style, extra fees the doctor might charge, or the time it takes to get an appointment with a specialist. When I hear these complaints, I am convinced that the difficulty lies in feeling uncomfortable in expressing concerns or dissatisfaction to the doctor or any other authority figure.

Some of you may feel intimidated by the doctor and don't want to say you don't understand or that you're upset about having to wait two hours, or perhaps you think that's just the way it's supposed to be. More serious concerns, such as waiting months to have a hip replacement or knee surgery, may well go unsaid because you think "Why rock the boat?" or "I don't want to upset the doctor." In essence, you might convince yourself it is not important to communicate how you feel; you'd prefer to keep the peace. Your reluctance to speak up may relate to your personality or the way you interact with others, or perhaps you feel you depend on the doctor. Cancer patients, for instance, may feel a higher degree of dependence than someone visiting the doctor for a cold. This can vary, of course, according to who you are as a person and what level of support you need and from whom. Deciding when to speak up can be a balancing act, especially when sharing how you feel with your family or general practitioner (GP) or a specialist, such as an oncologist. (**Note**: The terms family practitioner or general practitioner are used interchangeably within North America, but for the purpose of this book I will use the term GP for consistency reasons.)

Any number of factors can influence your degree of sharing. For example, communication may be easier with your GP simply because you might visit the doctor more often than you see your specialist so you develop a more relaxed rapport. However, if you have chronic pain or a life-threatening condition that requires you to meet frequently with a rheumatologist, an oncologist, or a psychiatrist, you might feel just as comfortable with him or her as you do with your GP.

For the purpose of this book, we will focus on how to communicate with your GP. However, some illustrations in the chapters ahead will include interacting with other health-care professionals or a health-care team, such as specialists or nurses. Many of the communication strategies can be used with most health-care professionals. Similarly, the examples you choose will reflect your personality or personal style. In fact, this is important because you want to sound as natural as possible in your communication. I cannot emphasize enough how important it is to bring a list of your symptoms to your appointment with your doctor. This is a great reference tool to keep matters at hand succinct and clear.

For some of you, the process can be awkward, even if you are communicating positive feedback. We all want the process to be smooth when we ask questions or express concerns to the doctor, whether it is about feeling rushed or about aches and pains. You might even want to thank your doctor for his or her support or treatment.

One thing to remember is that the discomfort level decreases with practice. One way to become confident in communicating on different levels with the doctor, or anyone for that matter, is to take action. You take action by visualizing or preparing what you want to say in your mind or by writing it down. You can rehearse it with a good friend. You can say it out loud in front of a mirror. When you do this, take a deep breath, exhale slowly, and listen to the tone of your voice, your words, and your delivery style. If saying it out loud is too difficult, consider writing a note or letter. It is important to recognize the impact of your words and style on your doctor as well as understanding how the doctor's style affects you. Once you understand this, you are in a better position to take ownership of your decision-making powers about your health care.

Part of taking ownership of your health care is to discover and understand how our health-care system works and who can help us keep well, work toward recovery, or leave this world with dignity. Chapter 1 addresses this multileveled structure and its benefits and downfalls. In the remaining chapters, we will examine specifics of how to communicate with your doctor. Throughout the book I've included examples drawn from the stories I collected when I was researching the book, and wherever possible I've tried to capture their spoken words so you can "hear" different styles of communication and find the one that suits you best. The names are made up, but the cases are real, and the strategies are prolific. You'll also find checklists to help you evaluate your communications skills and your relationship with your doctor. Some of the questions seem to keep popping up over and over again — that's because as you learn more, your answers might change. Note that you can print the checklists and access the links in the Resources by using the download kit. The instructions are included at the end of this book.

Much of this book relates to communicating with the doctor, with suggestions along the way on how to understand yourself better or communicate on behalf of another on issues of health. Underlying this information is the principle that each of us has an ethical responsibility to take action on behalf of our own health care as well as to communicate pertinent information to the doctor that will assist toward your health improvement. Let's get started!

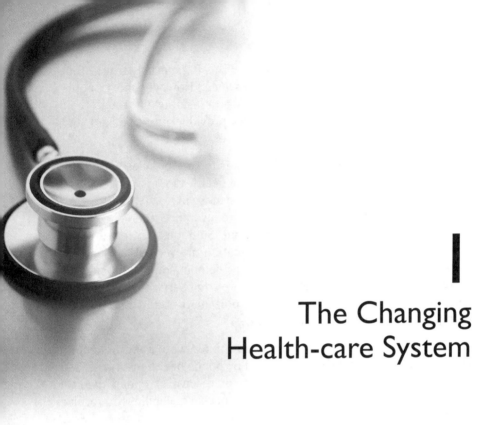

1
The Changing
Health-care System

Communicating within the health-care system today differs from five or ten years ago. The constant reorganization of hospitals and health-care delivery and changes in health-care insurance coverage have put a strain on health-care administrators, practitioners, and consumers. Whether it is within the United States or within Canada, each place of residence is experiencing similar challenges and shifts. Some of these shifts are positive and some are negative.

One of the effects of these changes is the shorter period of time that a person stays in hospital. Another is that health-care professionals can no longer give the amount of attention during a visit that they did five or ten years ago. Public and private health insurance no longer covers the same range of services it once did. Walk-in clinics are more frequently used, in part due to the fewer number of general practitioners (GPs) who accept new patients (this depends where you reside). In many instances, people who can pay out of their own pocket can move forward on a waiting list for some treatments, such as colonoscopy surgery. Someone who is unable to pay might have to wait in the line up, and he or she may be there for months. (This is especially true within Canada, and varies from province to province.) However, most people do have some form of extra or private health insurance (through their employer or by paying a health-insurance provider out of pocket), and that is important in today's medical culture.

For certain, with the onset of new health-care policies within the United States, everyone *must* have private health-care insurance. There is also public health-care subsidization for those in North America with low income. If you do not have health-care insurance, then check with your local Royal College of Physicians and Surgeons or Health Maintenance Organizations (HMO) for information or even ask a friend for names of health-insurance providers. For comparison sake, I suggest gathering at least three names to compare what services are provided and for how much. Take note, it is important to read the fine print within any insurance policy document.

There are options, however. A consumer who wants extended care, that is, more care than is covered by public health insurance, can purchase private health-care insurance or receive extended medical coverage as part of an employee benefits package. People who receive social assistance or a pension are entitled to special medical and drug benefits. I would suggest checking online for the specifics for your location.

Overall, the face of the North American health-care system has changed in recent years and it will continue to change. Within the context of these changes, each government health body anticipates improved health care for its residents. Some services will remain the same; and some will be replaced by new technology. No matter what, doctors and allied health professionals, such as nurses, physician assistants, physiotherapists, and dietitians, will remain constant in their service to you, the consumer. The system also aims to provide prompt care to those who need it, whether in an emergency situation or when a condition takes a dramatic turn for the worse.

In today's health-care system, you play a large decision-making role in your health care. This requires your cooperation and ability to communicate your health-care needs and wants. Asking your doctor, gathering written information, and talking to others are good ways to start.

Knowing about the various components of the health-care system is another good idea. The choice of medical facility is sometimes the responsibility of the patient. For example, someone in the city must decide if it is more appropriate to drive across town or go to a nearby walk-in clinic. It's better for a woman in labor, for instance, to go to the hospital than to a walk-in clinic. In some places, such as rural areas, the only choice might be going to an emergency department or medical clinic, or having a personal midwife. Of course, knowing the location of medical facilities is especially important in order to choose the correct facility for the situation. Regardless of where you see yourself in the overall scheme of things, you need to have an idea of how the health-care system works in your overall area.

Knowing what Medicaid covers and what extra health-insurance packages you need for your purposes is crucial to your care as well. It will be up to you to do some research on these matters; however, the Resources at the end of this book include websites that will help you explore different areas and increase your knowledge about what best suits your needs. You might want to ask your doctor if he or she can recommend resources. Your workplace might have health-care insurance add-ons where your employer will match your contributions taken from your paycheck. If you are on social assistance, there are health-care provisions that are available to you. Research what these are for your particular area and situation. The message here is: Be prepared.

1. General Practitioners

General practitioners (sometimes referred to as family practitioners) are the central link between specialists and allied health professionals. They are also the keepers of medical records. Their offices are like a holding tank for all the patient's medical records accumulated over time from other health-care professionals. GPs, along with specialists are expected to make sure patient records are detailed and organized so their colleagues can have easy access to the information. Most hospitals today also have a secure medical electronic system where most specialists can access their patients' information. Along with this, GPs, as with all doctors, must keep on top of their patients' medical histories, stay informed about new medical research, and run a cost-effective business.

Most certainly, the high expectations placed on especially the GP contribute to a demanding schedule, leaving less time for the doctor to spend with the patient. It's a good idea to keep a record of each visit with your doctor, along with a record of medications prescribed, and any blood tests results, whether you are a patient or a caregiver. The more you can keep on top of your own care, the more you encourage a healthier health-care system.

2. Hospitals

Hospitals are experiencing substantial changes. These changes affect the operation of the hospital as well as how you and the medical staff interact with each other. Such interactions can be demanding at the best of times.

The lengthy wait times has been consistent over time, primarily because of a shortage of staff or an overflow of patients. This is a North American phenomenon, especially with our ever-changing health-care system. It is partly due to increasing populations, stressed out society, and money allocation to different health services (some receive more money than others). It is also because patients sometimes choose to go to the hospital emergency rooms for small ailments such as the sniffles or minor scrapes when a walk-in clinic or a visit to the family physician might be a better and more efficient choice. There are also e-services that people can access via telephone or online within certain jurisdictions.

Similarly, the level of activity elsewhere in the hospital ebbs and flows. People are admitted for short term or long term, and doctors and visitors come and go. Nurses, even with their changing work shifts, are a constant presence — they are present in the middle of the night, and all day long to attend to a patient's needs. Other allied health professionals, along with doctors, make scheduled rotating visits.

In addition to providing care for people who stay overnight and outpatients, the hospital is also an administrative body that serves the community. It is supported by federal and state or provincial funding supplemented by large community donations. Some hospitals or allied health-care services are privately or partially privately funded and/or owned. Its board of directors and committee members make serious decisions about its operation. Considerations of federal and state or provincial guidelines and support play a very important role in its infrastructure.

In addition to those guidelines, hospitals are like any other institution that must follow certain rules. The staff has a mission to provide excellent care to the community in which the hospital resides, based on respecting the patients and employing professional health-care providers.

We should expect the hospital to honor its mission statement. Likewise, we should respect the hospital's true purpose, which is to care for the sick, not those with scratches or scrapes. A more appropriate venue for minor concerns would be your neighborhood community walk-in clinic or general physician.

3. Walk-in Clinics

Walk-in clinics are different from GPs' offices. Doctors at walk-in clinics usually work on a rotational basis, sharing the patient load with other doctors; therefore, people may not necessarily see the same doctor each time. Nurses sometimes assist with intake by reviewing the patient's concerns before the patient sees the doctor. Walk-in clinics are usually located in neighborhoods or communities, rather than in hospitals or medical centers.

People go to walk-in clinics for various reasons. Some may not have a GP or family physician. Some may need or want immediate attention. Some people might use the clinic as a regular medical facility for their care, or they might not be able to find a doctor taking new patients. Many are transient patients who don't return to the same clinic. Whatever the reason, the doctors at walk-in clinics often treat people with symptoms of common colds, allergies, or minor scrapes. More serious ailments are redirected to a specialist in a private office or hospital setting.

In this example, Eric chose to visit a hospital for symptoms of athlete's foot. He waited two hours to see a doctor, and then, during the examination, the doctor reprimanded Eric for inappropriate use of a medical facility.

Eric's choice was not well thought out. He would have received more immediate attention at a 24-hour walk-in community clinic. His waiting time would likely have been shorter and he would have received treatment right away. The doctor would have determined quickly if Eric needed further attention at a hospital. This would have been a more efficient use of the health-care system.

4. Health-Insurance Plans

There are differences and similarities between the American and Canadian health-care systems. Both systems provide a provision for those employed to purchase or pay into a private health-care insurance policy as well as to purchase private and additional health-care packages outside of the workplace. These vary according to your place of residence. Some family physicians might be willing to recommend health-insurance companies to you; while others will not feel comfortable with this. Some insurance companies will provide limited or wider-scale coverage. This is up to the patient to examine the fine print and then make a decision as to which package is best for him or her.

In Canada every person is entitled to health-care services supported by public funding. This public funding comes from Canadian taxes. It is a myth that all services are provided through public funding alone. In more recent years, if patients want faster service, they will pay out of pocket for it or have extra private health insurance to cover the costs. For instance, should a doctor recommend an MRI for discomfort in the abdominal area, and the wait-list is anxiety inducing to the patient, the patient is not prohibited from seeking a medical imaging facility that will accept an out-of-pocket payment for an immediate or fast-tracked MRI.

Health care in Canada is based on a simple proposition: Every legal resident is covered through a publicly financed provincial or territorial plan. The individual mandate, derived from a Republican precedent in Massachusetts, stands in stark contrast to Canada's universality principle. Even though Obamacare broadens coverage, the individual mandate relies on a fundamental insurance principle — care depends on type of coverage — and compels Americans to purchase insurance to access care. Americans now have more affordable insurance options and subsidies to cover their costs, and the lowest-income may be eligible for public coverage through the expansion of Medicaid. Still, despite the crush of online traffic as enrolment began, only half of the estimated 40-plus million uninsured will be affected by Obamacare.

5. Ambulatory Care

New technology has made ambulatory care an alternative to inpatient care. It is based on efficient and simple day procedures. By removing overnight care, hospitals can reduce their costs. Most people are content to use ambulatory care services, primarily because it avoids an overnight stay in the hospital.

6. Home Care

Home-care programs also decrease hospital care, allowing people to remain in the comfort of their own home. Home-care programs provide support services such as assessment and case management, home-care nursing, physiotherapy, occupational therapy, homemaker services, along with helping people bath, cut their toenails (foot care in general), and so forth.

Many of these short-term services are provided by nurses, reha-bilitative, therapeutic, and assistive home health care. This care is pro-vided by registered nurses (RNs), licensed practical nurses (LPNs) or registered practical nurses (RPNs), who work with home-care agencies. These services help adults, seniors, and pediatric clients who are re-covering after a hospital or facility stay, or need additional support to remain safely at home and avoid unnecessary hospitalization.

7. Meals on Wheels

The Meals on Wheels service delivers meals to individuals at home who are unable to purchase or prepare their own meals. The name is often used generically to refer to home-delivered meals programs, not all of which are actually named Meals on Wheels. Because these people are housebound, many of the recipients are the elderly, and many of the volunteers that deliver the food door to door are also elderly but able-bodied and able to drive vehicles, usually a van. You can find the Meals on Wheels chapter in your area by searching online. Of interest, Meals on Wheels is also in many other countries around the world.

8. Palliative Care

Palliative care offers people with terminal illness treatment to make them comfortable by helping with symptom and pain management, of-fering counseling, and meeting their basic needs. Starting in 2006 in the United States, Palliative Medicine is now a board-certified sub-spe-ciality of Internal Medicine with specialized fellowships for physicians who are interested in the field. Within the Canadian health-care system there are privately and publicly owned medical facilities that provide palliative care. Like other components of the health-care system, these programs are supported by state, provincial, or territorial federal fund-ing and private donations.

The palliative care patients who reside in these facilities range in age; they can be children, adolescents, middle-aged adults, or seniors. The facilities are staffed by doctors, nurses, nurses' aides, dietitians, nutritionists, social workers, spiritual counselors, and volunteers who work together to meet the needs of the patients. The services can be provided through nursing care and other support services, and there are day programs offered by volunteer services. There are even 24-hour response teams available for emergencies or short-term support. In addition to palliative care provided through a home-care program, various types of facilities offer palliative care, such as the following:

- **Long-term care facilities**: Nursing homes and hospitals usually have palliative care services for those needing long-term care. People with Alzheimer's, for example, may reside in long-term care for up to 12 years, if not longer.

- **Hospitals**: Some hospitals set aside a certain number of beds to meet the needs of those needing palliative care; other hospitals may have an established palliative care unit with a team of specially trained health-care professionals.

- **Hospices**: A few residential hospices exist in North America. These are houses or apartment buildings where palliative care is provided in a home-like setting. Some people use their palliative care service on a 24-hour basis.

Palliative care presents a challenge to caregivers because the terminally ill person often has difficulty communicating. Family members or friends often speak on the person's behalf. In such a situation, the person's needs or wants should be expressed in a living will, or a power of attorney should be granted to someone who will act in the best interests of that person. It should be emphasized that a patient should appoint a caring, communicative individual for this role while he or she is still cognitively aware. Nevertheless, a professional and highly rated palliative care unit will have staff trained to identify the needs of the patient.

However, some people are very capable of communicating their needs and wants to staff and caregivers. For example, Reba's dying mother, who was living in a long-term care facility, wanted to speak with a pastoral care counselor. A staff member arranged for the pastor from Reba's community church to visit with her mother every week. Reba's mother could have requested a monthly visit, but she felt a need for more regular visits.

Whether people are able to communicate or not, palliative care employees recognize that the primary needs of the patients are comfort, kindness, and professional health care. Meeting these needs requires time and appropriate lodgings. Obtaining the right facility at the right time is not always a given. Waiting for a bed for an ill relative or friend can be frustrating, particularly if you prefer a specific facility. Access to this type of facility depends largely on available space and financial resources. The cost of this service can vary and sometimes paying out of pocket is the only solution.

A good place to start researching appropriate medical or financial resources for palliative care is your family physician or community care access programs. You can also get information from specialists, home-care nurses, social workers, pastoral counselors, seniors' groups, community clinics, the library, or friends. Look in the phone book or on the Internet for other information sources, such as American or Canadian Hospice Palliative Care Association, Cancer Society, and AIDS Society within your respective countries.

9. Other Community-Based Programs

Community-based programs provide assistance and attention to people who are at risk. The services are offered by doctors, allied health professionals, and trained community volunteers who make every effort to care for those most in need and often unable to fend for themselves. They also lift some of the weight of responsibility from the shoulders of caring families, unable to cope with doing it alone. In addition, most of these programs provide access to valuable resources, such as drug plans.

Doctors, public health nurses, or counselors work in clinical care, as do some trained volunteers. Community-based programs often include patient education, preventive health care, prevention against diseases such as sexually transmitted diseases (STDs), community programs for new mothers, regulations, and vaccination centers across North America.

Trained community program planners, public health nurses, child and youth workers, and others provide community-based health programs for children and youth, First Nations communities, and rural and community health programs. It is the rural areas, however, where these resources are most lacking, unfortunately.

9.1 Mental health care

Mental health professionals, such as psychiatrists, psychologists, social workers, and nurses work in a hospital or community-based setting. They work with children and youth, violent offenders, substance abusers, and dementia patients as well as other mental health problems and disorders. That said, this is another, and serious area, of the health-care system in North America that is burdened with long waiting times for those needing these services. It can take up to three months to a year to have a patient connected with a mental health professional for out-patient care or in-patient care within a hospital setting.

Sometimes there are walk-in community care centers where a person can access a limited time (six weeks, possibly) with a mental health worker, but again this depends on the wait times. Universities and colleges usually have mental health workers available on campus for students. The student must approach the campus medical center for a referral.

9.2 Pharmacare

Pharmacare is a system of subsidization for prescription and non-prescription drugs. Drugs include prescription medicines and over-the-counter (OTC) medicines such as for cough and cold, and personal health supplies (e.g., oral hygiene products or diagnostic kits). The doctor prescribes the medicine, the pharmacist dispenses it, and the individual receives it in the hospital or in the community. For the most part, over-the-counter medicines and personal health supplies are pur-chased in drugstores and paid for by the consumer. Prescription drugs are paid for by many payers — governments, hospitals, private insur-ers, employers, and unions as well as people paying out of their own pocket. Except for drugs received by people in institutional care, drugs are not always covered by the *United States National Health Care Act* or *Canada Health Act*. Some North American locations have federally subsi-dized drug programs for specific groups, such as First Nations people, veterans, seniors, and social assistance recipients.

9.3 Virtual medicine

Virtual medicine, sometimes referred to as telemedicine, provides an-other means of accessing health-care services and advice. The services are accessed from the Internet or through telephone e-health care ser-vices set up around the world (see Chapter 8). It is used in both the medical and dentistry fields where it has several advantages over con-ventional systems. We know virtual reality is used in surgery, especially in the field of robotic surgery where it has proven to be very successful.

Virtual medical clinics are now international, ranging from family physician advice to sports medicine information. There are virtual sites where the patient can communicate face to face with a health-care provider via the Internet. The physician and patient can see each other, and if necessary, the patient is able to show the online physician a medical condition such as a rash to assist with diagnosis.

Accessing health care online is becoming a more common experience, especially for those who might not have a family physician. There are also those who like to surf the net to gather additional information about a diagnoses they were given by their family physician, or to gather more precise information about a set of symptoms they have to bring along with them to a doctor's appointment.

Whatever the reason for accessing information — whether it is virtually via a website or in-person with a health-care provider — the way in which you communicate and what you do with this information is a big part of how much you will benefit from it. It is always recommended that you check with a health-care professional that you know to verify the validity of the information you gathered or received. In this day and age there are always online and off-line scammers wanting to make a fast buck at the expense of a vulnerable person. So, be safe with your personal information and learn more about the advice you receive from others.

10. The Health-care Team

Almost all health-care services involve health-care teams. Health-care teams are an integral part of our system. They exist in hospitals and privately funded facilities as well as include your general practitioner (GP). Each member of the team has specific duties, yet each one shares the same objective, which is to ensure the patient's progress. Some of the teams involve different medical services, such as oncology (cancer care), gynecology, general medicine, infectious disease control, and surgical teams. By linking together to achieve optimum diagnosis, treatment, and support care, these health-care teams offer a substantive service.

At a teaching hospital, which is affiliated with a medical school, the health-care team generally consists of interns, residents, the attending physician (who is usually a specialist, such as an oncologist), and medical students, along with allied health professionals such as physician assistants, registered nurses (RNs), registered practical nurses (RPNs) or licensed practical nurses (LPNs), social workers, psychiatrists, psychologists, pastoral care counselors, pharmacists, dietitians, and nutritionists. The attending (faculty) physician is responsible for the ultimate decision-making for patient care, and supervises medical care for specific services that he or she oversees.

The medical student on the health-care team is in the early stages of his or her education. Each student is assigned a few patients, primarily to follow up with them. Their primary goal is to learn patient care, and they also report to residents or interns, fill out reports, and write details on a patient's status.

The intern is a recent medical graduate. Interns are more involved with medical services, such as checking lab reports and tests. They collect information about a patient's status and follow up with patient care.

Residents are responsible for making decisions in the absence of the attending physician. They may be required to lead the team for a specific medical service, such as oncology.

Fellows are medical doctors who are working toward extra qualifications in a particular specialty, such as in gynecology. Their decision-making powers lie between those of the resident and those of the attending physician.

Consult teams are sometimes put together to give advice or treatment for a particular specialty. For example, if someone who has had a kidney transplant is having problems, a renal consult team might include a nephrologist (kidney specialist), hematologist (blood specialist), a nurse who specializes in dialysis, and a social worker.

Allied health professionals are health-care workers other than doctors who have special training in the performance of supportive health-care tasks, such as nurses, social workers, and nutritionists, depending on the needs of the patient.

Regardless of the time of day, the team members meet to discuss various cases in an attempt to diagnose, but also to learn. Then they do their rounds, which means as a team they visit patients in their rooms. For example, when Sam's father, Eduardo, was hospitalized with a bleeding ulcer with heart complications, the medication for his heart condition aggravated his ulcers, causing massive bleeding. His condition worsened within a couple of days and he developed serious pulmonary problems. Eduardo was not expected to live. His health-care team was a standard one: The resident visited him periodically throughout the day, and a nurse regularly checked his vital signs and bedside intravenous tubes connections. As Eduardo got closer to dying, the specialist worked with Sam and his family to prepare for the event. When Eduardo finally died, a nurse stood by in the room as a presence for the family until the priest arrived. Each team member aimed to make Eduardo's last moments as comfortable as possible.

Although primary health-care groups resemble a team, team members do not necessarily work in the same physical environment. Primary physicians (GPs) or family physicians (FPs), for example, are usually linked to other caregivers, such as a cardiac specialist, a dietitian, or other health-care professionals. For instance, when a patient called Ron complained to his GP about chest pains he was sent for an immediate cardiogram, but also was referred to a cardiologist.

Communication between the GP and the cardiologist was likely by telephone, email, or computer fax system on behalf of the patient. In similar circumstances, a patient's medical record or test results are shared among the primary health-care team, ensuring a greater understanding of the person's condition. (Patients sometimes need to verify with the specialist that the GP will receive this information since automatic transference of records varies according to location.) Sometimes, depending on the distance, physicians will consult with one another by Skype.

Health-care teams work as a system, sharing balance of care. They exist in many formations, within different medical services, as with palliative care teams, psychiatric care teams, and general medical teams. You, as the consumer, have this team available to you, no matter what your condition. You are entitled to the attention of the member of the team who can offer you the best support for your needs, whether you are the patient or caregiver. To make the most of it, though, it is up to you to ask and tell the team your concerns. You must also bear in mind that each team member has a specific role. If you ask a question and you are referred to someone else, you are not being brushed off — you have asked something that is outside that person's jurisdiction or expertise. Make sure you understand the responsibilities of the team members.

The Royal College of Physicians and Surgeons in North America are governing bodies that develop policies to ensure that physicians provide ethical care to any and every patient. It is this body of people that a patient can email a complaint against a doctor's inappropriate or unethical behavior (e.g., physical or emotional abuse).

11. The Limitations of the System

When Tom made an appointment with his ophthalmologist because of failing vision in his left eye, the only appointment available was four months away. His wife, Sandy, waited three months for an appointment with her GP. When she arrived for her appointment, she was told her doctor was on maternity leave for five months. Sandy's appointment was with a replacement, or what is referred to in medical speak as a "locum." Sandy was surprised that she hadn't been told beforehand, especially since she had called that morning to confirm her appointment. She ended up seeing the locum but was frustrated because she didn't feel comfortable with a stranger, and because she didn't feel she had much choice, since she had waited so long for the appointment, and didn't know of any other doctors accepting new patients.

Tom and Sandy compared stories. He had been annoyed when he had to reschedule his appointment for four months later — having already waited four months. His doctor's medical office assistant said the reason was that the doctor had to attend to an emergency. Apparently, there were no back-up specialists, and the assistant did not even try to find an earlier opening for Tom.

Unfortunately, Tom and Sandy's experiences are similar to those of other health-care consumers who are frustrated by delayed or postponed appointments. People often feel they have no alternative since finding another doctor can be difficult, leaving little recourse for unhappy patients. Sometimes it seems as though the changes made to the health-care system have put limitations on the delivery of health care in North America. Overall, the sense of limitations creates a domino effect, ensuring the medical community and consumers feel there are growing barriers to care.

Even with some increased enrolment rates within medical schools, there is a new attitude of those medical graduates. Some newly graduated family physicians are not so fast to set up a practice of their own. They are quite happy to work on-call for physicians taking a vacation or a break from working. For example, Maria, who is a university professor, crossed paths with a former undergraduate student. Pleased to see him and hear that he now had the title of Medical Doctor, she asked him where his new practice was setup. He gleefully said that he was not planning to set up a practice just now since he could work as often as he wanted as a locum or on-call doctor and still make enough money. He said he didn't want the stress of a practice, allowing him also to have freedom to travel in between interim work. Maria nodded in agreement with his thoughts but wondered how that fared for the patient really needing care in an already challenged medical care environment. It is also a challenge for doctors already overloaded with a patient roster. They are most definitely overburdened with an aging population. In some hospitals, the reduction of full-time nurses is forcing doctors to take on more work or shifts to make up for fewer staff.

In the case of Emily who works as an LPN in an obstetrics unit, she has been expected to fulfill duties that only doctors or an RN once had the privilege to do. In her specific case, she is now expected to take blood samples from a patient and send it to a lab. The paperwork involved in recording some of these newly assigned roles takes up the time from actually working for the patient. With such a stressed health-care system in North America, and added responsibility, it leaves room for errors in patient care. This certainly leaves food for thought for the patient wanting better care. It also leaves health-care professionals frustrated because they want to give good care.

The following are possible barriers to patient care:

- Patients' reluctance or inability to express their concerns and frustrations.
- User fees for certain services (e.g., transfer of medical records, written medical certificates).
- Long waiting lists (e.g., for appointments, emergency departments, elective surgery) due to shortages of appropriate staff (e.g., specialists, GPs, technicians) and hospital beds.
- Time constraints on doctors to see more people in less time.
- High costs of drugs and technological equipment.
- Changes in services covered by health-care insurance plans.
- Funding cuts to hospitals, home-care programs, etc.
- Approval time required for public access to drugs or for coverage by health-care insurance companies.
- Approval time from health maintenance organizations for paid services.
- Overworked staff in hospital settings.

- Mismanagement of medical funding.

- Mismanagement of health-care facilities and services.

- Poor physician communication of important patient facts relevant to their care.

- Poor patient communication with the health-care provider, such as information sharing.

The following are continuing and new supports for care:

- Subsidized medical services within North America.

- Public funding within Canada.

- Availability of home care, if needed.

- Availability of palliative care and spiritual support according to individual faith.

- Availability of a variety of community health-support groups.

- Newly accessible health-care services for Americans with the onset of the Medicare program.

Although there are benefits to the overall North American health-care system, we do need to learn how to maneuver around the limitations that prevent us from getting optimal health care. Don't be discouraged — the new medical culture will bring more improvements. Already we are seeing new drugs designed to slow down growth of cancer cells or reduction of memory loss in some dementia diseases. New technologies are allowing for quicker and more defined diagnoses. Home care is allowing patients to remain in the comfort of their own homes. Programs such as Meals on Wheels give those who are housebound opportunity for good healthy meals. Part of what makes the health-care system better is well-informed patients who know how to use the system to get optimal health care. That's why it's important to take action, be assertive, and communicate on behalf of your own or someone else's health-care needs. See Checklist 1.

Checklist 1
Do You Know What's Available?

Check either yes or no to the answer that most relates to your knowledge of health services and facilities available to you in your area. Review your answers to these questions and assess any gaps in your knowledge or your care. What steps will you take to improve the situation?

Question	Yes	No
Have you recently moved to a new neighborhood, state, province, or territory, or country?		
Do you know where the nearest hospital is?		
Do you know how to get to the nearest hospital by vehicle or public transportation?		
Is the hospital a teaching hospital?		
Does the hospital have ambulatory care or outpatient services?		
Does the hospital offer services in languages other than English?		
Are the hospital services satisfactory to your needs?		
Do you need to be close to a hospital with services for children?		
Do you know if there is a professional home-care service available for the elderly?		
Is there a walk-in clinic close to you?		
Do you have a reliable general practitioner (GP)?		
Does your GP have an on-call service or replacement when he or she is not available?		
Does your GP have hospital privileges? (This depends on where you reside.)		
Does your specialist or surgeon have a separate office outside the hospital to treat patients?		
Does your GP make home visits or return telephone calls within 24 hours?		
Do you know what fees your GP charges for such services as copies of medical records, transfer of records, or issuing medical certificates?		
Do you require a night nurse, social worker, pastoral care, or palliative care?		
If you are in the hospital, do you understand the roles of various members on the health-care team?		
Does your doctor (whether in the GP's office or in the hospital) take time to discuss your concerns?		

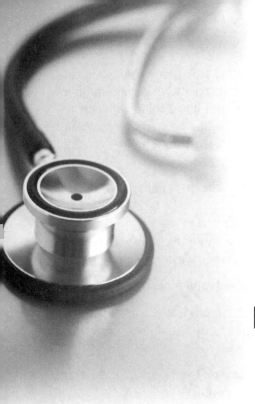

2

Knowing Yourself

Our response to being a patient can depend on our age, gender, culture, health, personality, lifestyle, experience, and ability to communicate. These factors make up who we are and how we interact with others.

Your health can affect the way you interact with others. For example, if you're not feeling well, you might be unpleasant and surly, or you might be whiny and passive. Perhaps you're obstinate and uncooperative when you're under the weather, or maybe you become especially dependent on others. At the doctor's office you might want a hint of nurturing, or you might be impatient for the doctor to assess your condition quickly. Whatever your particular style, your response to the state of your health influences the way you communicate your symptoms.

Let's look at some different styles. Lilith's response to being ill is to make a concerted effort toward getting well. When she visits her doctor, she clearly communicates her impression of her symptoms. After they have an open exchange about the possible prognosis, she readily accepts her doctor's recommendations. As a patient, Lilith is assertive and co-operative. She is also willing to take a proactive approach to her health care, and works with her doctor to arrive at an agreeable treatment.

When Roland feels ill, he is grumpy and scowls at his wife and children. Like a pet that hides when it's sick, he creates a wall around himself. Roland refuses to go to the doctor until it's absolutely necessary, but as soon as he arrives in the doctor's office he starts to complain. In addition, he resists taking any advice, at least until he has had time to think about it.

An interaction between Roland and his doctor might go as follows:

Doctor: "What can I do for you today?"

Roland: "I don't know. I feel kind of achy all over. My wife sent me here. I didn't want to come. I told her it was a waste of time."

Doctor: "How about I check your glands and blood pressure first?"

The doctor examines him and finds he has a mild case of the flu. She recommends that Roland drink plenty of liquids and take a few days off work to rest.

He balks at the idea of taking any time off from work. "I knew coming here was a bad idea," he says. "Gee, do I have to?"

Roland's response to his doctor's advice is ambivalent; he might or might not take her advice. First he needs time to process the information before he makes up his mind. Roland's interaction style is resistant.

Tomas becomes very dependent when he's ill. He wants support from his doctor. His tone and body language tell his doctor that he is handing over the decisions about his treatment to him. He asks the doctor to check all his vital signs, for reassurance, and then he accepts his prognosis without question.

Katie makes a list of all the things she wants her doctor to check as well as a list of recommendations for treatment. She tells her doctor what she wants and then asks for confirmation. She likes to make the choices about her health, with assurances from the doctor. Her style is decisive and informed.

Jetya visits her doctor once a year for a routine annual checkup. She is a recreational athlete who often participates in triathlons. She reads health and fitness magazines, along with updates on sports medicine. Her style of interacting with her doctor is laid back and casual. For example, when her doctor leads off by asking how she is, she might answer as follows:

"Very well, thanks. No complaints, I am just here for my regular checkup. Life has been good these days. How are you doing?"

The doctor and Jetya might continue their casual conversation during the examination. Their rapport is pleasant, without any demands made on each other. Jetya is confident in the doctor and trusts him.

Because our backgrounds and influences are many, some of us might be comfortable with a more formal relationship with our doctor than Jetya's casual style. Culture can play a part in determining our preferences. Gender can also influence how we choose to interact with the doctor.

Hanan comes from a culture where having a male doctor is prohibited, in part, because she is female. The rules within her culture dictate that only a female doctor can see her. As a patient, she is not permitted to explain her symptoms; her husband takes on this role. A patient coming from another cultural background may be quite direct in voicing her opinion, taking a more proactive role in decision making.

Juanita is shy and passive, particularly in the presence of a male doctor. Now that she has a female doctor, she is quite talkative because she feels less awkward explaining her symptoms to someone of the same sex. She has gained confidence in her choice of a health-care provider.

1. Know Your Body

Part of being a healthy person is having a healthy body. That means being knowledgeable about what keeps you mentally and physically balanced, and what's normal for you. Maintaining this balance means eating a healthy diet and exercising moderately as well as keeping a record of your medical history.

Jacko is self-assured and knowledgeable about his body. He also keeps an account of his medical history, including medical facts about his family. When he visits his doctor he discusses the methods he uses to keep fit. Jacko knows his body well, and because he stays informed on medical research, he has a good range of medical vocabulary that helps him describe symptoms. Jacko's doctor is impressed with his interest in keeping healthy.

"I wish more of my patients took the time to reflect on how to maintain their health," she says. "When did you become so interested in knowing more about how to keep fit?"

"It started when I was an adolescent, long before you became my doctor. I was overweight, had trouble breathing, and basically sat around a lot. I never got any exercise. The other kids always teased me at school," said Jacko. "After my dad died of a heart attack, I begged my mother to stop feeding me. She got worried and took me to see the doctor."

"What happened next?"

"Our family doctor was really helpful. He got me to talk about my feelings, and then he started giving me advice. He made some suggestions, and I started reading books and magazines about keeping healthy. I got my eating habits under control and started to get involved in sports," said Jacko. "You know, that doctor really helped me change the direction in which my life was going."

"You have done well," said his doctor. "Here you are at 40 healthier than some 25-year-olds I've seen!"

Jacko grinned. "Thanks, doc."

Each of the people I've described in this chapter takes a different approach to their health, some more intense than others. The common denominator among them is that they all visit their doctor; this in itself tells us that on some level they care about their health.

For some of us, paying attention to our bodies comes naturally; for others, it requires more work and concentration on being healthy. See Checklist 2.

2. Know Your Communication Style

There are many different communication styles that can affect the interaction between you and the doctor. How you take in and process information is a basis for how you send and receive information.

As patients, we can communicate with the doctor better if we can identify the elements that contribute to our communication style. Knowing how we absorb and communicate information helps us make sure our wants and needs are met.

2.1 Gathering information

Let's start with looking at how we take in new information. Most of us acquire information through listening, reading, or seeing how things

Checklist 2
What Kind of Patient Are You?

Check yes or no for the answer that best describes you. Keep these responses in mind as you consider your role in your health care.

Question	Yes	No
Are you aware of the state of your health?		
Do you try to stay informed about the latest health treatments?		
Do you take your health for granted until there is a problem?		
Do you explain your symptoms clearly?		
Are you focused on your body's responses?		
Are you aware of how your body responds to stress?		
Would you describe yourself as a pleasant patient, as in cooperative?		
Do you make decisions easily about your health care?		
Do you depend on the doctor to make decisions about your health care?		
Do you prefer to have the last say in decisions about your health care?		
Do you feel comfortable asking your doctor for explanations and information about your health?		

work — or some combination of all three. Although we usually prefer one over the other, the three methods can complement one another.

For example, George needs to have information explained to him before he is able to understand its true significance. This doesn't mean that George cannot process information in any other way; it just means that he understands more when he hears it. As a patient he listens attentively to the doctor's explanation.

Karina processes information most effectively by reading. For her, the written word is concrete evidence of information; it is right there in front of her. As a patient, she prefers to read a brochure or pamphlet rather than listen to spoken instructions or explanations.

Samuel, however, is able to have a deeper understanding of information by being shown a picture. As a patient, he understands best when his doctor illustrates his explanations with diagrams or models.

George, Karina, and Samuel might use all three methods of gathering information, but only one is their preferred means to understanding and retaining new information. See Checklist 3.

Checklist 3
How Do You Gather Information?

Check the answer that best describes you.

Question	Yes	No
Do you gather information best through hearing?		
Do you gather information best through seeing pictures?		
Do you gather information best through reading?		
Do you often ask for explanations from your doctor?		
Do you carefully consider the medical information you receive?		

2.2 Perceiving, organizing, and interpreting information

How we perceive, organize, and interpret information from the doctor influences our response. Simply said, our beliefs, values, and attitudes affect the way we understand. These are learned through family and societal influences. Our emotional state also plays a role.

Let's say your doctor tells you to take a long break from working because you are suffering from exhaustion. If you perceive this information as a negative reflection of your job performance, you could interpret this advice to mean that you are a failure. Your emotional response to what the doctor says may cause you to become very upset with the doctor. But what if you have a different interpretation? You might organize the information you receive in a different way and come up with a different interpretation. You might agree with the doctor's prescription for overcoming exhaustion.

Suppose, in another instance, you feel your doctor does not seem to understand your symptoms accurately. You try to clarify the information, but still there is a misunderstanding. You might decide that the doctor is being obstinate and unwilling to hear what you have to say. Perhaps you are right; however, the doctor's ability to understand is affected by the way he or she feels that day. If you can figure out the real reason for the misunderstanding, you might be able to get your message across.

How might you do this? You could remain objective and explain that you feel that you are not getting your point across. You could say, for instance, "Doctor, for some reason I don't seem to be describing my symptoms clearly. I wonder if there is some other way I could describe them". If you say this, the doctor has an opportunity to recognize that perhaps he or she is misunderstanding you. You also have stepped back from the situation and checked your own perception. You've had to listen to yourself as well as to the doctor.

As you can see, how you respond reflects how you choose to process what you have been told. Of course, processing information includes other behavior that makes up the success or failure of your communication approach. Let's look next at listening.

2.3 Listen to yourself and the doctor

Listening can play a primary role in keeping well. It involves hearing, attending, checking, understanding, remembering, and evaluating. Many people take this process for granted. We might think we are listening because we hear what is being said, but sometimes we are not registering the information. For example, we might tell the doctor about a symptom and we might hear what the doctor says, but we don't absorb what we are told so we don't follow the advice. Perhaps we are reacting to how the advice is being given, or we don't believe the advice is valid.

Sometimes, of course, we fail to listen to our symptoms of tiredness or ill health. We forget that we can't always function at full tilt all the time. Listening to our bodies is an essential part of staying well. For whatever reason, we may not yet be ready to listen to others or ourselves.

2.4 Attending to information

The depth at which we pay attention influences what we do with the information received. For instance, if we think the doctor's advice to lose weight is just a routine warning the doctor always gives out, more than likely we would make no effort to do so, and the consequences would probably result in more health problems.

Jill, for example, visited her doctor with complains of increased tiredness. The doctor observed that her tiredness might be a result of a weight gain during the previous year.

"Jill," said the doctor, "I see from your medical chart that we had this conversation six months ago. Did you follow my advice about eating a more balanced diet and getting more exercise?"

"I tried," answered Jill, "but I just can't seem to find the energy to do it."

"What have you tried doing?"

Jill frowned. "I tried walking every day for a week, but it was just too hard."

"You just have to exercise more and eat better, Jill," said the doctor sternly. "Then you'll have more energy."

This scenario obviously shows that neither doctor nor patient is attending to the other's concerns. Jill offered no information that might explain why she is unable to improve her diet and exercise more. The doctor didn't ask any questions about Jill's lifestyle that might offer insight into Jill's inability to take charge of her health. However, if the exchange was more like the following, the outcome would be different:

"I have been so tired in the last while," said Jill. "So tired that I find it difficult to even take a walk."

"How long have you felt this way?" asked the doctor.

"I think it's been about six months."

"How far have you been trying to walk?"

"I was trying to walk for forty minutes a day," said Jill, "but I only managed it for about a week."

"Perhaps you could start with a ten-minute walk for the first week or two," suggested the doctor. "That would be less tiring. Then you can gradually increase the time to twenty minutes. Within a few weeks you will be able to walk for forty minutes."

"That might work," said Jill. "But I'm so tired all the time. I'll give it a try."

"Good. Why don't you book a follow-up appointment in about two weeks so we can see how you're doing? We can take a look at creating a food plan for you then."

In this scenario, Jill and her doctor have allowed for more than one perspective. In doing so, they have paid attention to each other. Jill's reference to walking showed a willingness to attend to her health concerns, but her answers to the doctor's questions revealed she needed more information about starting an exercise routine. The doctor explored Jill's difficulty with sticking to a balanced exercise program.

2.5 Paraphrasing

Paraphrasing, or putting what you hear into your own words, is a large element of good listening. It's also a good way to check that you accurately understand what you're being told. By paraphrasing and checking your perceptions you can avoid frustration and misunderstanding, which reduces the time it takes to get the proper diagnosis and treatment.

For example, 36-year-old Lea had an active life before she became plagued with chronic pain and low energy levels. She was no longer able to participate in sports and other recreational activities with the same enthusiasm. She persistently sought advice from experts in conventional and alternative medicine. She also read numerous reports on a number of chronic pain diseases. Lea and her husband visited at least 25 of these experts, to no avail. Medical reports described her as neurotic as well as a noncompliant patient. In turn, Lea described the health-care professionals as being equally difficult. It appeared that they were at an impasse.

Eventually, Lea found a GP who diagnosed her condition as fibromyalgia, which involves chronic sore muscles, tiredness, and mental fogginess, along with other unexplainable symptoms. Because the doctor was aware of the severity of other symptoms, he took extra time to coach her on how to reduce her discomfort. After all her dealings with health-care professionals, by now Lea had learned to paraphrase and make sure she understood everything she was told.

"Doctor," she asked, "could you please repeat to me what I can do to make myself more comfortable?"

"Sure," answered the doctor. "First, make sure you stretch before you exercise. You might also want to reduce the intensity of your exercise regime for now to see how your body responds. I don't mean that you should stop altogether, but slow down for now. Another thing to do is reduce your caffeine intake." He handed her some brochures. "Here's some more information you can read when you get home, and we can talk about it some more at your next appointment."

"Okay, let me get this straight. I should take some time away from my regular sports activities, which are fairly intense. I should change some of my eating habits and then I should report back to you on how I'm doing. Right?"

"Right, Lea. Your next appointment should be in two weeks."

"Will that be my last visit for a while?"

"No, I think I should follow up with you for the first while until you feel comfortable with supporting your own routine," said the doctor. "Of course, we can discuss other approaches, too. The goal is for you to be able to make these changes on your own."

"I think I understand," said Lea. "You will follow up with me regularly to check how I'm doing, and you'll help me develop strategies to take care of myself."

"Yes, I'll guide you toward developing new ways to manage your condition. There are all kinds of options to explore, such as attending support groups, and there are some good books and articles on fibromyalgia. For now, start with those brochures I've given you. There's lots for you to learn."

"That's great, but it won't take me long to get through them!" said Lea. She was impatient to know more about her condition. "Maybe I could check the bookstore on the corner, or the library for some of those books."

"There are lots of places to get good information," said the doctor. "Ask at your pharmacy, too; many drugstores have DVDs and books on different conditions."

Do you see how Lea repeated what she was told in her own words? She was checking her perceptions, and reinforcing the information she received. She was also practicing active listening, which improved her communication skills.

If we are mindful listeners, especially in patient-doctor exchanges, we will experience better results. We can observe how the information exchanged with one another affects both parties in the exchange. By listening carefully, we acknowledge others and ourselves.

Keep in mind that information is sent and received as a transactional process, a process of give and take. So while you listen to the doctor, the doctor is also "listening" to your response by seeing you nod or make gestures and by watching your eyes and face for reactions. It is a back-and-forth process that focuses on the verbal and nonverbal patterns of communication. The outcome of the exchange reflects how well we listen.

2.6 Listening too hard

Some listeners analyze every word or phrase they hear. They have to consider the information extra carefully in order to understand all the bits and pieces. They might be cautious in their interpretation of new information and listen especially closely in order to evaluate a recommended treatment. For example, Marisa tends to over-examine any condition related to her health.

On her last visit, her doctor said, "My medical office assistant tells me you are concerned about a dry skin patch on your arm."

"Yes," said Marisa, holding out her arm. "It is here."

The doctor examined the skin. "It looks like a flare-up of eczema."

"A flare-up; does that mean it's really bad?"

"Oh no, it's minor," replied the doctor. "Nothing a little medicated cream won't help."

"Are you sure, doctor?"

"Yes, Marisa. This is not very serious."

"What about that red spot?" Marisa asked. "It looks bad, and it's very itchy."

"I've seen a lot worse. Don't worry, I'm sure it will clear up with this cream." The doctor opened a drawer and took out a sample tube of cream. "I'll give you a prescription, too."

"Why do I need a prescription, too? Do I need two kinds of cream?"

"No, this sample isn't enough to last you more than a couple of days, but you need to apply the cream two or three times a day for at least a week. The prescription is for the same cream."

"How do I know if I should apply it twice or three times?"

"If the skin is still red and itchy, apply it three times a day," the doctor explained. "You can go as high as four applications, but only apply a little at time. You don't need to slather on huge amounts. But when it starts to be less uncomfortable, then you can apply it twice a day. "

"Okay," said Marisa uncertainly. "I think I read somewhere that eczema is infectious. Maybe I should have been more careful."

"No, not to worry. It's not infectious; you can't catch it from other people, and you can't spread it by touching someone. It's just an inflammation or irritation of the skin," said the doctor. She handed Marisa a pamphlet. "This has some more information that might help."

"If it's not infectious, how did I get it?" asked Marisa. "Maybe I'm worrying too much!"

"That's all right, Marisa, these are good questions," said the doctor, trying to reassure Marisa. "Eczema can be caused by many things. It could be your laundry detergent or it could be stress. Read the pamphlet and try the cream for a week. Then come back and we'll take another look at it."

Marisa appears to need to pick apart everything the doctor says until she arrives at an answer that satisfies her. It is her way of looking after herself. However, her persistent analysis is sometimes overdone. How can Marisa take a more realistic view of what the doctor is saying?

She could listen more objectively to herself and the doctor. She would notice that her objectivity would make a difference in how she responds to the doctor's advice. If she practices her listening, she might discover she can assess information more objectively. This would probably make Marisa more confident in her interactions with her doctor.

2.7 Selective listening

At times we hear the information given to us, but we listen or process the information selectively. In other words, we choose what to pay attention to and block out the rest. This is not necessarily something we do deliberately. This sometimes happens when we are distressed by what we hear, such as when we are told upsetting news about a loved one. We try to defend ourselves against the effect of this information.

For example, a doctor tells two adults that their mother has bowel cancer, with a large tumor. He says that there is a 90 percent chance that its progress can be prevented before any real damage is done, but there are no guarantees until their mother can have exploratory surgery. Both people hear the doctor's statement differently.

The daughter heard that her mother had a 90 percent chance of recovery. The son heard that she had a lesion that was quite long, giving his mother little hope of recovery. Both people selected what information they paid attention to and evaluated, rather than hearing the actual meaning of what they had been told.

When we're confronted with very serious news, we might listen defensively for a couple of reasons: We don't want to hear bad news, or we prefer to hear the worst scenario to avoid disappointment down the road. Such responses may allow us time to adjust to the reality of such situations, but the result is often confusion later on.

There are ways to avoid the confusion. For example, we could ask the doctor to clarify what's being said. We might paraphrase what the doctor tells us. We could also try to remain objective, as difficult as this might be, and wait for more concrete results. What is crucial in similar circumstances is to listen attentively, instead of selectively. Any of these approaches will prepare you better for the outcome. See Checklist 4.

Checklist 4
Not Listening

Listening depends on a number of things, such as our physical capacity to hear, or our state of mind. If you are not listening, ask yourself the following questions.

Question	Answer
Are you stressed, preoccupied, or unwilling to listen? Do you know why?	
Do you understand what is being said?	
Does the doctor understand what you are saying?	
Are you overreacting to what is being said?	

Fred's experience is a good example of not listening. He had high blood pressure and a high heart rate, along with a quick temper. When his doctor suggested that Fred take a stress management program, he interpreted her suggestion as an insult. He became so angry that he got red in the face and started yelling at the doctor. Once the doctor was able to calm him and explain what stress management involves, he admitted that he needed some help. Fred's emotional state interfered with his ability to listen, preventing him from assessing his doctor's recommendations accurately.

Within this scenario, we see that many factors can interfere with listening. If the information is not received, then confusion is the result.

Listening also allows the opportunity to consider another point of view. Particularly in the area of health care, discussing other perspectives opens up possible solutions to problems, and this allows for a potentially healthier life.

2.8 Listening with memory aids

In all these examples the person receiving the information does not absorb what the doctor is saying. Often people need memory aids such as notepads, recording devices, or the like to absorb what is being said to them.

Whatever the reason, although the patient appears to be listening, the information does not register. Patricia, for example, cannot absorb information in an intense atmosphere. In that kind of situation, she feels dazed. For her, visiting the doctor is an intense experience. As a result, she does not clearly hear what he tells her. After she leaves the office, she realizes she doesn't know the exact recommendations the doctor has given her. On her last visit, she telephoned the doctor when she got home. He suggested that next time she bring a notepad with her, or ask a friend or relative to come along to help her review her questions or comments. The next time she went to the doctor, she took notes, and found that it helped her process the information the doctor gave her. This time she didn't feel so dazed! See Checklist 5.

3. Talk to the Doctor

Many people are not aware of how their own delivery style can influence the responses they receive from other people. People who communicate directly, for example, usually get right to the point of what they want the other person to hear. Someone who communicates non-directly might use "doublespeak" or might talk around the point, hoping that the listener will figure it out. These communication styles encourage various responses.

Checklist 5
What Kind of Listener Are You?

Check yes or no to the answer that best describes you.

Question	Yes	No
Are you an attentive listener?		
Are you a selective listener?		
Are you a defensive listener?		
Are you a mindful listener?		
Do you paraphrase information?		
Do you check to make sure you've understood what you're told?		
Do you question information?		
Do you make sure you understand what you've heard before you speak?		
Do you evaluate information?		
Do you organize your thoughts before you speak?		

Let's say, for instance , that Joe said to his doctor, "Doc, I'll get to the point. There's a history of prostate cancer in my family and that's why I am here today. I want you to do an examination."

"All right, Joe," said the doctor. "Do you know what's involved in the exam?"

"No," answered Joe. "Explain it to me."

"Many men find the exam embarrassing," said the doctor. He explained to Joe what he was going to do. As he talked, Joe listened carefully and interrupted when he had a question.

"Will it hurt?"

"It won't be painful, but you will feel some discomfort at times. It doesn't last long, though," said the doctor.

Once Joe was satisfied he understood what the doctor told him, the doctor examined Joe. Afterward Joe said, "That was the most unpleasant experience I have ever had."

The doctor agreed. "Yes, I told you it's an uncomfortable exam."

"Yup, I can't say you didn't warn me. Good thing I knew what to expect!"

Joe and his doctor's open communication style allowed for a candid exchange. It also provided a defense against embarrassment or awkwardness for Joe, because Joe was able to talk about his feelings directly.

However, if Joe had an indirect communication style he might talk about everything else going on in his life before broaching the subject of a family medical problem. Finally, near the end of the appointment, he might mention that his father recently died of prostate cancer. He might express nothing more about his own fears about this disease. Although his doctor would recognize the seriousness of the statement and arrange for another appointment, there might not be any explanation of what Joe could expect, which could lead to confusion and misinformation.

3.1 Assertive delivery

An assertive communicator is usually confident and articulate. The delivery is polite, yet firm. Assertive communicators know what they want and are often skilled at delivery. In other words, when they are presented with a situation they feel strongly about, they don't hesitate to take a stand.

For instance, Yang's doctor wanted her to try a prescription drug for depression. Yang, however, felt strongly that antidepressant drugs would decrease her ability to fend off depression on her own. Her doctor explained that it would help her balance her mood, and that she could also try therapy. Yang, adamant that she would do it her way, articulately explained her own view.

"I understand your point, doctor," she said. "However, I think I'm strong enough to work out a coping strategy."

"Medication will help improve your state of mind," said the doctor. "I've observed that you've been depressed for a while, and the antidepressant will help lift some of the immediate stress."

"Don't you think it would be better if I use my own inner resources first?" asked Yang. "I've been reading about herbal remedies and the effects of exercise on emotions. I think there are healthier ways to deal with depression than through mood-altering drugs."

"You have a point," said the doctor. "But your depression has been going on for some time now. I really feel it would be to your benefit to at least give it a try."

"I want to try some of these alternatives first. For example, I haven't tried meditation or other stress-management strategies." Yang explained some of the methods she had been reading about. "If I find these other ways of coping don't work and I'm still having bouts of deep depression, then I will consider trying your way."

"Well," answered the doctor hesitantly, "that seems reasonable, but let's talk some more about these other strategies. I would like to see you every couple of weeks while you get started."

Yang delivered a reasonable alternative to her doctor's recommendations. She remained level headed, and pointed out sensible and healthy options for herself. She also guarded her preference for a non-medicated approach to dealing with depression, and she negotiated with the doctor that she would consider medication if she felt it necessary. This style of communication allowed for Yang and her doctor to compromise.

3.2 Nonassertive delivery

There are a number of reasons why you might not feel comfortable with some doctors but feel comfortable with others. You might feel shy about talking about your body or your emotions with someone of the opposite sex, or even of the same sex. You might not know how to identify or describe what you're feeling, whether it's physical or emotional. If you're like Zita, you might not have the words to describe how you feel.

When the doctor asked Zita how she was feeling, Zita replied, "I'm not sure."

"Can you tell me what might be wrong?" asked the doctor.

"I don't feel well. Somewhere around here," said Zita, pointing toward her stomach. She sounded uncertain.

"What does it feel like?"

"It's hard to describe," said Zita. "It's just kind of sore."

"Is it your stomach?" asked the doctor. "Perhaps you can tell me what you've eaten in the last few days."

"Not much ... a little yogurt. That's all I could digest."

"Come over here to the examining table and let's have a look." After Zita laid down, the doctor began to do a routine check of her stomach. "How does that feel?"

Zita winced, but all she said was, "It's okay."

The doctor finished his examination, and said, "I think there's a little more acid in your stomach than usual." He went over to his desk and wrote something on a piece of paper.

"Here's the name of an antacid," said the doctor, as he handed Zita the slip of paper. "You can get it in any drugstore." He turned away to make some notes in Zita's file.

"Oh, okay," said Zita. She had a feeling there was something more she should tell the doctor, but she wasn't sure what.

Her doctor wondered why Zita came to visit him just for a minor stomach upset. Zita's nonassertive manner and limited description of pain gave the doctor little information to go on. His quick assessment of Zita also left her dissatisfied, but Zita seemed to be feeling too awkward to say anything else.

Why was this such an unsuccessful visit for both patient and doctor? The doctor did not probe more deeply into Zita's pain and took a poor history of her condition. Zita lacked good delivery skills for describing her discomfort. How could this interaction have been different?

The doctor could have prompted or guided Zita to describe her problem clearly. This could indicate the source or degree of the problem. Zita could have tried to identify her pain by trying to describe its location and how severe it was. It might have helped if she had thought this through before she arrived at the doctor's office. For example, she could have written a description, perhaps that the pain resembled a bruise or burning feeling. By defining her pain, she might avoid a repeat visit for the same complaint or, worse yet, a misdiagnosis.

It's not uncommon to feel shy about expressing your feelings to someone who seems to have more authority than you do. It is especially difficult for people who are afraid of the response of others.

3.3 Aggressive delivery

An aggressive communicator usually has a forceful tone and is unwilling to negotiate any point of difference. Aggressive communicators feel they are right and everyone else is wrong. Their style is to attack verbally and assign blame. Their strategy is usually to be overbearing, silencing the other's views, and their tone of voice is confrontational and sometimes angry. These kinds of communicators want to cut off the other person with demands. Their escalated emotional state makes it difficult to reason with them. Such a delivery style may get you what you want, but not without consequences. You might end up being asked to leave the doctor's office permanently!

For instance, Louie is late for every appointment he has with the doctor. When he arrives, he is usually rude to the medical office assistant, who must now tell him that he'll have to wait until the doctor can squeeze him in between the other patients who showed up on time. He mutters about having to wait, and then, once he gets into the doctor's office, he rants about the assistant's unwillingness to rearrange the schedule. During the exam, Louie rejects any suggestion the doctor makes. When he leaves, he slams the door behind him. The same thing happens every time Louie goes to the doctor, and every time everyone in the office is relieved when he leaves. Louie's aggressive style leaves everyone upset, plus it's hard on his blood pressure and detrimental to his health.

Louie goes through life like this, but there is a difference between someone who is routinely aggressive and someone who is aggressive on occasion. Jackson, for example, was upset when his shoulder injury forced him to take time off from recreational sports. His doctor had given him pain relievers for the persistent pain, and she recommended ice packs, whirlpool treatment, and acupuncture. Jackson used the medication but didn't bother with the other recommendations. After a couple of weeks, he still felt pain. When he went back to the doctor, he was furious. With a raised voice, he demanded to know why the medication had not decreased the pain.

"Have a seat," suggested the doctor. "Let's discuss this calmly."

"No," said Jackson angrily. "I want answers now!"

"I am not so sure that is going to happen if you speak to me in that manner," said the doctor firmly. "Maybe you should take a walk around the block and cool down first."

"What kind of lame response is that?" shouted Jackson.

"Jackson, you're clearly upset and in no state to discuss anything," said the doctor. "When you've calmed down a bit we can discuss your situation. Perhaps I should leave you alone for a moment."

Jackson began to realize that his feelings were out of control. "Wait a minute, doctor," he said. "It's just that my shoulder hurts just as much as it did before … "

Jackson and his doctor began to discuss his condition and why the drug might not have been effective on its own. In the end, Jackson apologized to the doctor.

"I'm sorry about that outburst," he said. "I guess I let my emotions run away. I shouldn't have taken it out on you."

Louie's and Jackson's approaches are both extreme. As we've seen in this chapter, there are many other aspects to communicating effectively. However, it's always important to take into account your own personal style as well as the doctor's style. For instance, you might be a high-spirited person, but your doctor might have a more reserved demeanor — this difference in style can contribute to potential misunderstandings.

Each of us wears many hats, so to speak, so choosing the best one for the occasion might create the best image. When you're in the doctor's office, it might be a good idea to remain neutral, polite, and even-tempered in your delivery of thoughts or complaints. See Checklist 6.

Checklist 6
What Type of Communication Style Do You Use?

Check yes or no for the answer that best describes you.

Question	Yes	No
Are you assertive?		
Are you shy?		
Are you direct?		
Are you aggressive?		
Are you confident?		
Are you compromising?		

By now, you probably have a sense of who you are and what your communication style is, along with basic delivery skills. Try practicing those skills in front a mirror, with a good friend, or simply reflect on your own communication style. Once you've refined your style, you can paint a clear picture of what you want and need.

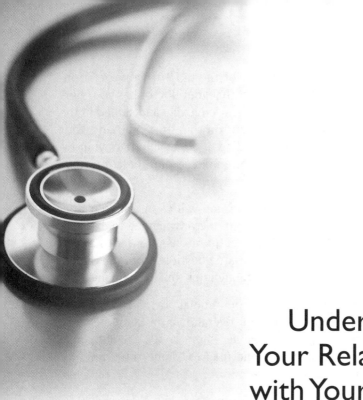

3

Understanding Your Relationship with Your Doctor

General practitioners are the central link between us and the rest of the medical community. They make referrals to specialists and allied health professionals, who rely on your GP to provide your comprehensive medical history. Likewise, your GP relies on you for a clear description of your family history and symptoms.

As mentioned in Chapter 1, the GP's workload is increasing. With heavier patient loads and more administrative responsibilities, the GP must still keep informed about the latest medical research. Governments, the community, and health-insurance providers are placing increasing demands on them. As a result the GP's decision-making role is intensified, and the GP has a greater effect on the quality of your health care.

1. Dependency and Vulnerability

Most of us have required a doctor at one time or another. Some of us see our doctor frequently, others not very often. The relationship you have with your doctor is possibly one of the most trusting relationships you will have in your life. You trust that your doctor has your best interest at heart and that he or she is knowledgeable and skilled in the practice of medicine. Because you count on this trust, you and your doctor must develop a good understanding of the dynamics of your relationship. These dynamics include different levels of interaction. Your trust might vary according to how ill you feel.

Nevertheless, at one time or another you will count on your doctor's diagnosis or advice. At that time your doctor will need to examine you physically or ask you deeply personal questions in order to assess your circumstances and needs. Appropriate questions from the doctor about your health are necessary, even though they might seem invasive.

For example, when Eta arrived for her annual physical, the doctor asked her a list of questions about her overall health. Some of these questions directly related to her lifestyle. She is a 30-year-old single professional who had been dating one man for some time. She has been seeing this doctor since she was 15.

The doctor asked, "How is your sex life these days?"

"Fine," said Eta with a smile. "How's yours?"

"Well … ," the doctor laughed. "The last time you were here you had just met a nice man. I gather you're still seeing him?"

"Oh, yes, it is going very well."

"Are you and your boyfriend having sexual relations?"

"Yes," said Eta. "That's going very well, too, thank you."

"Good, have you been using protection?"

"Don't worry," replied Eta. "You taught me well. As a matter of fact we decided it would be a good idea to have tests done for sexually transmitted diseases."

"I see," said the doctor. "I gather then that you both feel the relationship is moving in a positive direction."

Eta nodded.

"Then I think you have made a good decision."

In this case, Eta and her doctor felt comfortable enough to be candid with each other. Their interaction felt light, instead of intense.

Not everyone is as comfortable with these kinds of questions. Some people find such questions make them feel vulnerable and awkward. A similar scenario may then produce another response.

Sixteen-year-old Matty was scheduled for her first complete physical exam. After taking a detailed history of her health, the doctor said, "Matty, are you sexually active? We should discuss contraception options."

"Oh no," said Matty. "No, I am not. So I don't need any information."

The doctor noted that Matty seemed nervous. "That's okay," she said, "but I want you to feel free to talk to me if you need anything."

"Sure." Next the doctor began to explain what was involved in the rest of her checkup, and Matty seemed to understand.

"Here is a gown to change into," said the doctor. "I'll be back in a few minutes."

When she came back, she took Matty's blood pressure and pulse rate and then, as she had explained, she began to examine Matty's breasts. By the time she started the abdominal examination, Matty was clearly very tense.

"Are you comfortable with this?" asked the doctor.

"No," said Matty quickly.

"It's natural to feel uncomfortable, especially the first time. Do you want to talk about it?"

"No!"

"Why don't we do this another time?" suggested the doctor. "That will give you some time to get used to the idea of the physical exam. How about you book an appointment for six months from now?"

"Yes," said Matty, noticeably relieved.

When the doctor sensed Matty's discomfort, she tried to talk about it, but because Matty was clearly unready, she chose to postpone the examination. After six months, Matty might feel differently; it will ultimately be her decision. (By the way, most women and men of all ages feel uncomfortable with their routine checkup.)

Your doctor will likely adapt the tone and structure of the questions to how well he or she knows you as a patient. Depending on your age, the questions will remain along the same lines. If you are uncomfortable with personal questions, it is best to mention it to the doctor. More than likely, your doctor will understand.

2. Patient Expectations of the Doctor

Our primary expectation of our doctors is that they help us to get well and stay well. We also expect our doctors to have a reasonable amount of time to spend with us and we expect them to be able to communicate effectively. We expect our doctors to be in a good mood. Plus we expect our doctors to have answers to all our medical concerns.

If you ask people if these expectations are met, some will say "yes" but more will say "no" or "sometimes." Why are these negative replies so common? It may be that our expectations, which are often based on a stereotype, are unrealistic, or it might be the result of a breakdown in communication.

Remember Louie in Chapter 2? He expected the doctor to receive him immediately despite the fact that he arrived late for his appointment. Louie also expected his doctor to put up with his irate manner. Louie forgot, first, that the doctor had patients lined up before and after his own appointment. He also forgot that he deserves no more attention than do the other patients. For some reason, Louie's stereotyped view of a doctor is that the doctor is there to "serve" him on every level. This view is false; remember, the doctor is there to help you get and stay well.

In contrast, when Wendy visited her doctor for a cold, the doctor was annoyed with her for taking up valuable time for "just a cold." Wendy was surprised that he would speak to her in this manner. When he saw her reaction, he apologized for his irritability. He later explained that he had a heavy patient load that week and he was worried about his young daughter, who was sick. Wendy learned something new. She realized that her doctor had a point about a needless visit and that he too had personal and daily stresses.

A person's expectation of the doctor as the perfect caregiver often sustains the view of the doctor as having an air of mystique. How much "mystique" the doctor has varies among different age groups, societies, and cultures, and even between the sexes. Someone who comes from a culture where obedience is emphasized may hesitate to challenge the decision of a doctor. Someone in their 70s, for example, might be more compliant than someone in their 30s, although any one of us at any age might have this view.

For example, Elita, at 37 years old, was under the impression that doctors remain poised under all circumstances. When she told her doctor about her own emotional response to a situation in her life, she noticed the doctor's eyes filled with tears. It threw Elita off balance for a second, since she expected a doctor to respond differently from the way she herself responded. She was touched by her doctor's show of sympathy, and felt a little silly to be reminded that her doctor was, after all, human.

Today, much of this mystique is decreasing as people begin to speak more openly with their doctors. Because the talk is more open and frequent, the mystery about "who is this person I give so much authority to" is reduced.

Media images of doctors contribute to both the mystique and its breakdown. Some television shows, especially those on cable networks, add to the doctor's image as the mysterious figure whom the patient places on a pedestal. Prime time television often depicts emergency room procedures or the interchange between doctors in tense situations. In fact, many of those shows portray doctors coping with their personal lives and convey the message that doctors are as vulnerable as any of us.

This is not to say that television accurately depicts the life of doctors. But with some semblance of a doctor's personal life, people can empathize and identify with the doctor. To this end, our expectations will level out with new insights of the doctor as an ordinary person, not just a professional.

Nonetheless, some people don't want to think of their doctor as having another life. They might prefer to place the doctor on a pedestal. This might be the best way for them to feel safe in the hands of someone they have chosen to help them stay well. The point is that our expectations are varied, and more than likely they suit our purpose.

3. What Kind of a Relationship Do You Want with Your Doctor?

By now you have probably thought about what kind of relationship you have with your doctor. You might be perfectly happy with the services and the interpersonal exchange your doctor offers. However, you might have decided to change the quality of this relationship, in which case there are a few considerations to keep in mind.

Ask yourself what kind of relationship you want with your doctor: Do you want it to be dependent? Independent? Aloof? Friendly? Consider whether you and your doctor have similar attitudes and values about health care.

3.1 Attitude considerations

Lara felt she had a generally good relationship with her doctor except that she felt frustrated by a lack of feedback when she expressed concern about some health matters. Her doctor sometimes brushed aside her questions and moved on to something else. Lara felt her doctor's attitude in this situation was aloof.

On one occasion Lara asked about her headaches, which kept recurring. The doctor replied, "It's nothing to be concerned about. Just a little stress."

"But they're so persistent and they're so painful," said Lara. "Maybe I need to have some tests done."

"If you rest, it should help," the doctor said, without looking up from writing in Lara's medical file. "Now is there anything else that you are concerned about?"

Lara felt it was futile to press the issue. She ended up suffering in silence.

Lara wondered whether this attitude reflected her doctor's overall approach to her health care. She needed to decide if it was worth addressing this with the doctor. How would she approach her? She discussed it with her friend, Ellie, who was a nurse.

"I'm not sure how I should to talk to my doctor without sounding confrontational," she said. "I mean, she might see this as an affront."

"Are you second-guessing how she might respond?" asked Ellie. "She might be more receptive than you think."

"She seems so aloof. Maybe I should say something like 'Doctor, I feel when I tell you about my headaches that you don't take me seriously.' I can say this without sounding threatening. This way she might see it as a real concern."

"She might take it more seriously if you make a special appointment with her," suggested Ellie. "However, what if she responds in the same aloof way as before, or if she gets upset?"

"I'm not sure." Lara thought for a moment. "I'll have to decide if the doctor's attitude conflicts with my own attitude."

"Then what will you do?"

"Well, there are a couple of options, I guess. I could ask for a referral to a specialist. Or I could find another doctor who will take me a little more seriously."

"That sounds like a good plan," said Ellie. "It might be hard to find a doctor taking new patients. I know mine isn't!"

"There's that walk-in clinic down the street," Lara said. "Someone told me the other day that he found his doctor by asking at the hospital if there are any recently graduated doctors looking for new patients."

"Another place to search would be on the Royal College of Physicians and Surgeons website for your area," said Ellie. "I hope you can work out something with your doctor. You know, this discussion reminds me of a situation my brother had with his doctor."

"Oh?" asked Lara. "What was that about?"

"Values, I think."

3.2 Value considerations

In order to trust your doctor, you need to feel that you share the same values, as we see from the following story of Ellie's brother.

"You know how my brother Toby was recently diagnosed as being HIV positive? When his doctor called him in to inform him, Toby said his attitude seemed different," said Ellie.

"What gave him that impression?" asked Lara.

"Toby said his doctor seemed more serious, less interactive in a way. He wouldn't look Toby in the eye."

"Maybe the doctor just felt bad for Toby," suggested Lara.

"That's what Toby thought at first," said Ellie, "but then the doctor said something that made him rethink the doctor's response."

"What did he say?"

"He told Toby that he could no longer be his doctor and that he was referring him to a specialist who would then refer him to another GP."

"Maybe he didn't feel he knew enough about the condition to continue as Toby's doctor," said Lara.

"Toby asked him that," said Ellie. "He said no; he just felt that Toby would be better off with another doctor. That's the only explanation he gave."

"Hmmm, sounds like he's uncomfortable with Toby."

"That's what I think," said Ellie.

"I guess he felt there was something different about Toby and that was what made him uncomfortable."

"Maybe he thought Toby is gay, and he's uncomfortable with that. Wouldn't you think he'd discuss that with Toby?"

"That would certainly be the professional thing to do," said Ellie. "It's not like Toby hasn't been his patient for a long time! He didn't even discuss with Toby how he might have caught the virus".

"Sounds like he judged Toby without finding out the facts."

"The interesting thing is that Toby later found out he'd been infected by a woman who's HIV positive. At that visit, the doctor wouldn't even talk about it. He didn't have the integrity to tell Toby how he really felt. Toby didn't realize the possible implication of the doctor's decision until later."

"Toby never asked the doctor to explain his feelings?" asked Lara.

"No, but what difference should it make? Toby shouldn't be judged either way."

"True," said Lara, "and if that doctor has a problem with stereotyping specific groups then your brother is better off with a doctor who has different principles."

"You are so right, Lara! That's exactly the way I feel. I guess he could have made an official complaint but he figured he would just move on."

"I bet most patients don't know what their doctor's views are on those kinds of things until some situation arises. My doctor's values might be completely different to mine."

3.3 Behavior considerations

Ellie knew another story about someone whose behavior interfered with his relationship with his doctor.

"It's just not different values that can make dealing with the doctor awkward," Ellie told Lara. "I remember this one person I worked with when I was a nurse at a community health center. This had more to do with the patient's behavior."

"What happened?" Lara asked.

"This man arrived expecting to see the same GP he usually saw, but when he got there he discovered that the doctor was on holiday. The man got really upset and started yelling about how that doctor was always on holidays and that he was slacking off on the job."

"In front of everyone in the waiting room?" asked Lara.

"The receptionist knew it would be disruptive for him to be out in the open like that, so she guided him to a room and sent me in to calm him down. He ranted and raved for a good half an hour."

"How awful! I'd have shown him the door."

"I wish I could have!" said Ellie, shaking her head. "This man had absolutely no empathy for the doctor, and no respect for the others in the clinic. I let him go on for a bit and then managed to talk him down till he was calm enough for me to take his blood pressure."

"How old was this man?"

"It doesn't matter if he was young or old!" said Ellie. "No one of any age should behave that way. Can you imagine if a doctor just lost it like that? The Royal College of Physicians and Surgeons would hear about it in a flash!"

"I never really thought about the doctor's side of things," said Lara.

"Doctors can't behave like that, so why should the patient? Although I think nowadays a doctor can refuse to see a patient who is completely obnoxious. I mean really, it is just a matter of mutual respect."

"I guess each of us really has to participate responsibly in our own health care," said Lara, "and that means remembering that mutual respect is a big part of our dealings with the doctor."

4. Be an Active Participant in Your Health Care

One way to be an active participant in your health care is to get rid of any unrealistic expectations. Identify what you want from your doctor. Realize what it is you are prepared to do as an active participant. Then review whether your attitude about your own health care needs changing.

4.1 Taking action

The most important things in actively participating in your health care are that you take steps to take care of yourself and you communicate clearly and honestly with your doctor. Live a healthy lifestyle — eat well, exercise, and get proper sleep (eight hours a night). Describe your symptoms as clearly as possible. Educate yourself about any conditions you might have so you can talk with your doctor about any changes that might have occurred. Discuss the benefits and disadvantages of alternative medicines versus conventional medicines with your doctor. Develop a sense of whether you and your doctor think along the same lines in terms of approaches to health care. Basically, you are looking for some common ground between you and your doctor in terms of attitudes, values, and behavior. See Checklist 7.

Checklist 7
Do You Take an Active Role?

Check yes or no for the answer that best describes you. This checklist can help you decide if you and your doctor have similar ideas about health-care communication.

Question	Yes	No
Do you feel comfortable talking to your doctor?		
Do you feel your doctor is comfortable talking to you?		
Do you prefer to share decision-making with your doctor?		
Are you more comfortable with leaving decisions up to your doctor?		
Do you prefer your doctor to explain your health problems?		
Do you prefer to know only the bare facts about your health problems?		
Do you prefer a reserved interaction style with your doctor?		
Do you prefer a candid interaction style with your doctor?		

4.2 Educating yourself

Seeking more information than what your doctor has provided can help you toward a speedier recovery after any illness or surgery. Nelson, for instance, recently had open heart surgery and is following a routine program to improve his strength. Although he has been following up with a specialist, he also checks in with his GP. Nelson has been busy with his assigned program but as soon as he was able, he started gathering information about other programs. His enthusiasm in discovering more about preventive health care impressed his doctor.

At their first meeting after surgery, his GP asked him how he was doing. "Everything is going very well, thanks," replied Nelson. "I've started going to the gym three times a week."

"Did you just start exercising on your own?" asked the doctor. "Has the specialist been giving guidance with your exercise program?"

"Yes, I checked with him and the physiotherapist at the rehab program I was in," Nelson said. "I also took out some books from the library and spent some time looking on the Internet for information about exercise programs for cardiac patients. I also walk twice a week, too."

"Good for you, Nelson."

"I've been making some changes to my diet as well," Nelson continued. "The cardiologist suggested some low-fat cookbooks and I've reduced the amount of fat I eat."

"Sounds like you're on the right track," said the doctor. "Have you made any other significant lifestyle changes?"

"As a matter of fact," said Nelson, "my employer offered me a buyout so I've decided to take early retirement. I've even started painting again."

"I didn't know you liked to paint," said the doctor. "What kind of things do you paint?"

"I do watercolor landscapes. What with all this free time I've got, even with that stress management group I joined, I've got enough finished paintings to hold an exhibition."

The doctor laughed. "Let me know when you hold that exhibition. I'd love to see some of your work. You've made some good decisions about your lifestyle and health, and your blood pressure seems fine."

"Is there anything else you feel I should be doing?" Nelson asked.

"Just keep an eye on your responses to the medication and keep up with the exercise program. Remember, don't push yourself too hard."

"I almost forgot," said Nelson, pulling a piece of paper out of his pocket. "I have this list of questions to ask myself about how to be more involved in my health. I wanted to go over them with you."

"Good idea, Nelson. Let's have a look."

Nelson handed the doctor the list, and they went over each question.

"Nelson, I'm very impressed with the way you've taken charge of your health. May I keep this list? It might come in handy with some of my other patients. "

"Sure!" replied Nelson, looking pleased.

"Good. Thank you. You seem to be doing very well. How about coming to see me again in a month?"

"Sure, doc. I'll see you then." Nelson's efforts to look for activities beyond the ones his doctors suggested paid off for him.

He took time to research and asked for advice when he needed to, and he followed up with his doctors. By doing so, he committed himself to being an active participant in his health care. Checklist 8 includes the questions he asked himself.

The first time Nelson asked himself the first eight questions he answered "no" to seven of them. This gave him an idea of what he needed to change. A month later, Nelson asked himself the same questions again and added the three final questions (see questions 9 to 11). This time Nelson answered "yes" to 9 of the 11 questions, so he was able to assess his progress.

4.3 Avoiding taking action

In contrast, 30-year-old Beau has not yet reached the same level of awareness about his health as Nelson has. As a result he avoids a healthy lifestyle as well as ignores his doctor's advice. Recently he returned to his doctor's office with a painful arm and a negative attitude.

"Beau, why are you back so soon?" asked the doctor.

"My arm is still bothering me a lot."

Checklist 8
Are You an Inactive Participant?

Check yes or no for the answer that best describes you.

	Question	Yes	No
1.	Do you listen to your doctor's advice?		
2.	Do you listen to your own advice?		
3.	Do you take time to relax every day?		
4.	Do you get enough sleep?		
5.	Do you eat a balanced diet?		
6.	Do you exercise regularly?		
7.	Do you look after your hygienic needs?		
8.	Do you make an effort to take care of your health-care needs?		
9.	Do you take time each day to resolve worries and then put them aside?		
10.	Do you have a hobby or recreational activity?		
11.	Do you research ways to add to improving your health?		

"Did you take the prescription I gave you when you were here a week ago?" asked the doctor, looking at her notes. "I see I also recommended trying hot and cold compresses. Didn't those make it feel better?"

"No," said Beau. "I lost the prescription note. I tried the compresses for a couple of nights, but they hardly helped so I gave up."

"I'm not surprised your arm is still bothering you if you haven't followed my advice."

"What do you mean?" said Beau testily. "I followed your advice! I just couldn't get the pills."

"Well, now that you're here, let's take a look at some of these other issues we discussed. Have you started any kind of program to lose weight and quit smoking?"

"Well, no, doc," said Beau, uncomfortably. "I haven't been sleeping very much lately and I am so rushed at work. My arm has been killing me. It feels like there's never any time to look after myself."

"I think we need to talk a bit more about your lifestyle." She described different methods for quitting smoking, and then began to explain how his eating habits were affecting his health. Beau began to understand how the choices he made contributed to how he felt.

"Here is a list of foods I want you to start eliminating from your diet," said the doctor. "Come back and see me again in a week."

"What about the pain in my arm?"

"I think that the muscular inflammation has gone down now, so I don't think you need that prescription any more. Start using those hot and cold compresses again. They'll make a difference."

"Okay," said Beau. "Isn't there something else I can do?"

The doctor smiled. "Yes, Beau, the first thing you can do is take a more active role in caring for your health. The second thing is, if you can't listen to yourself, then listen to my advice. Are you interested in doing this?"

"Yes, I think so. But I might need help."

By the time Beau left his doctor's office, she had convinced him that she could only help him toward a healthier lifestyle if he was self-motivated. He agreed to follow her guidance as well as try to make an effort to change some of his poor lifestyle habits.

Both Beau and Nelson have a candid communication style with their doctors. Their doctors also take an interest in their overall well-being. It seems that Beau and Nelson are a "good fit" with their doctors.

5. Are You and Your Doctor a "Good Fit"?

By now you've probably evaluated whether your doctor is someone you can rely on or not. Perhaps you're confused at this point about how you feel. Before making any big decisions, you might want to consider more information or strategies for taking action.

Jasmine wondered whether she was a good fit with her doctor. At age 40, Jasmine was feeling so tired all the time that it began to affect her work and recreational activities. She had a history of low hemoglobin so she thought that her tiredness might have something to do with it. When she brought up the subject with her doctor, she did not like the response she received.

She described the scenario to her sister-in-law, Joanne. "I am not sure if I should look for another doctor or not. It seems every time I mention my concerns about being tired my doctor just passes it off as due to my age."

"Didn't you tell me recently that your periods have been lighter than usual?" said Joanne. "Did you mention that?"

"Yes," answered Jasmine. "I asked if my low hemoglobin had anything to do with it, but she just said, 'For your age it's normal to feel a bit sluggish.'"

"Did you tell her how stressed you are at work?" asked Joanne.

"No, I didn't say anything about work. Do you think I should have?"

"Well, maybe if she had that information she might have assessed you differently," said Joanne.

"Yes, but don't you think she should ask me those questions herself?" said Jasmine. "She made a judgement without probing at all. Your doctor doesn't do that, does he?"

"No, we usually spend quite a long time talking about what's going on in my life," answered Joanne. "He always asks me if anything is different."

"That's what I think a doctor should ask!" said Jasmine. "Mine hardly talks to me and never shows much interest in what I have to say."

"Sounds like you're thinking about finding a doctor with a different manner."

"Yes, I am," answered Jasmine. "I won't give up mine yet; not until I find someone new."

"What are you going to do in the meantime?"

"I think I'll make another appointment to see my doctor and ask to see a specialist," answered Jasmine. "If she responds positively, I'll have to reconsider my decision. After all, I probably have to be a bit more assertive with her."

Jasmine's personal expectations of her doctor were valid for her. Her decision to discuss her frustration with a friend was useful because it helped her see her circumstances objectively. What's important in this story is that Jasmine decided to take steps toward changing the situation, whether it meant staying with her doctor or moving on to someone whom she felt offered a more compatible approach to her health care.

Cora, in contrast, was satisfied with her 25-year relationship with her doctor. She had entrusted him with the delivery of her three children through to treatment for her menopausal symptoms. She described their relationship to Jasmine.

"There were plenty of times that he was there for me. When Joey was little he used to climb all over things — once he fell off the table and landed on his head. I was frantic! I called the doctor and he squeezed us in right away," Cora said. "Then, on his way home that night, he dropped by the house to see how Joey was doing."

"Isn't it too bad doctors don't make house calls anymore?" asked Jasmine.

"I'm telling you, we have a terrific relationship. I know I can turn to him. He made time for me two years ago when my husband suddenly died. He made sure I looked after myself and he took care of my physical health, but he also always gave me the time of day."

"It sounds like you and your doctor have a really good relationship."

"Yes, it's been very satisfying. Now he's getting ready to retire, and I just don't think I'll be able to find another doctor who I can trust as much as I trust him," said Cora. "I'm sure he's going to find a good replacement, but it'll mean starting over with a new person who won't know me as well as he does."

Jasmine and Cora have different needs. In some respects both leave the decision making about their health care up to their doctor. Jasmine was more doubtful and needed more assurances, but she also wanted to be heard. As a result, she re-evaluated her situation. Cora knew her concerns were heard by her doctor and in turn she respected his recommendations, so she felt no need to question their relationship.

Often we don't consider the quality of our patient-doctor relationship because we don't think we have a choice in the matter. We do have some choice in its quality by knowing how to evaluate and communicate our needs.

There are pros and cons to every relationship and the patient-doctor relationship is no different. If there are more pros than cons on your list, then more than likely you have a good fit.

If there are more cons, then you may want to take a second look at what might be wrong in the relationship. Is there any room for improvement? If not, you might have to start looking for another doctor who suits your needs better. In Checklist 9, check "yes" to the statements that best describe your relationship with your doctor. Add up your checkmarks for each column. Keep in mind, though, that no situation is perfect. Being reasonable and realistic about your demands is crucial.

Checklist 9
The Pros and Cons of Your Relationship with Your Doctor

Pros	Yes	Cons	Yes
Your doctor is an open communicator.		Your doctor is a poor communicator.	
Your doctor is willing to consider your opinion.		Your doctor is not interested in your opinion.	
Your doctor is respectful.		Your doctor perceives your opinion as a challenge.	
Your doctor has a sense of humor and/or pleasant manner.		Your doctor is sarcastic or flippant.	
Your doctor keeps organized medical files.		Your doctor keeps disorganized medical files.	
Your doctor has a cordial staff.		Your doctor's employees are unfriendly or rude.	
Your doctor does not make you feel rushed.		Your doctor makes you feel rushed.	
Your doctor keeps you waiting no more than 45 minutes.		Your doctor often keeps you waiting longer than 45 minutes.	
Your doctor keeps informed of recent medical research.		Your doctor does not keep up with recent medical research.	
Total of Pros		**Total of Cons**	

Today, doctors might be more preoccupied with their workload than ever, so your doctor might not be able to spend the time with you that you want. You have complementary choices for where you can turn for health care. There are community resources such as nutritionists, acupuncturists, or physiotherapists who can address some of your health-care concerns.

Remember, you have to take responsibility for building the patient-doctor relationship. As we've seen, this means asking your doctor questions about your health and knowing what kind of patient you are. As in any relationship, you should also make sure there is two-way communication between you and the doctor. Checklist 10 will help you assess your relationship with your doctor.

Checklist 10
Do You and Your Doctor Have a Good Relationship?

Question	Yes	No
Do you feel comfortable talking with your doctor?		
Do you need someone to communicate to your doctor on your behalf?		
Do you prefer a doctor who encourages preventive health care, such as exercising and eating a balanced diet?		
Do you prefer a doctor who offers alternatives to getting well other than by using medications?		
Do you prefer a doctor who is receptive to your impressions of your health?		
Do you prefer a doctor whose culture is similar to your own?		
Have you appointed a power of attorney to act on your behalf if you are too ill to make decisions?		

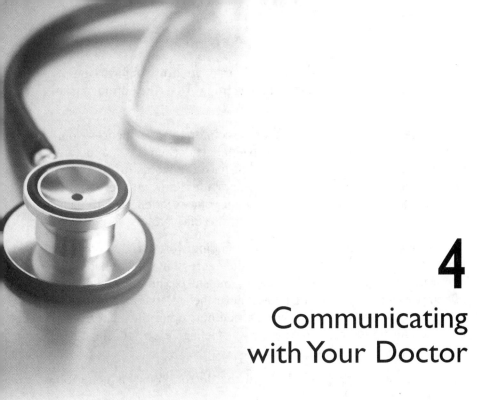

4
Communicating with Your Doctor

Communicating with your doctor involves exchanging information. In order for this exchange to be successful, both of you must understand what the other means. This means you must share a common language, which allows you and the doctor to clarify the information about your symptoms and arrive at a treatment plan.

1. Finding a Common Language

Finding the words and images that describe how you feel physically, mentally, or emotionally is difficult for some people. We often have our own set of expressions for describing these feelings; for example, some people think in words and others think in pictures. Just as we saw in Chapter 2, where people take in information in a variety of ways, some people prefer to draw a picture of their pain or discomfort; others are comfortable expressing themselves in words.

However, before you can express any pain, you must know exactly where it is and how much it hurts. Is it in your side? Near your hip or your groin? Is it deeply uncomfortable, or is it mildly uncomfortable?

What words or images describe the depth of your discomfort? Does it throb, or does it burn? Is the throbbing strong? Does the burning make you think of the color red?

The immediacy of the pain or discomfort also influences your choice of words and images. If that painful headache was there before your visit to the doctor, you might not have the words or images to describe how severe it was. Other factors affect how you respond to that pain, such as your age or attitude, or your experiences with pain. Your self-awareness and emotional state also play a role.

For example, Hannah has difficulty finding words to describe her emotions. She is at a loss to describe the depression she has had for a number of months. It is clearly a feeling, but she has no way of defining or comparing it in words. She knows, nevertheless, that on some level her depression is worsening. She reached out to her doctor for help, but when he asked how and why she was feeling depressed, she could not give a reason.

"You appear very sad," observed the doctor. "What is going on with you these days?"

"I'm not sure," said Hannah. "I've never felt this way before … at least not at this level."

"What do you mean by level?"

"Well … deeper, I think."

"Deeper?" asked the doctor. "How deep do you mean? Can you give me an example?"

"Do you mean like a hole in the ground?"

"Yes," said the doctor. "How would you compare the level of the way you're feeling with the depth of a hole?"

"I never thought about it this way." Hannah thought for a moment. "I think about two meters; just a little above six feet deep."

"That's interesting," said the doctor. "That's quite a deep hole. Let's talk about how we can help you with your depression."

At one point in their discussion, the doctor asked for other words Hannah might use to describe her feelings, and she talked about a deep, dark pit. The use of these images helped Hannah and her doctor draw a visual image of the depth of Hannah's depression. Her acceptance of the doctor's assistance gave her some insight into how to describe her feelings as well as helped to guide the doctor toward appropriate treatment. When her doctor asked her how she was feeling in a follow-up visit, she said she associated her feeling happier with the words "sunny yellow."

1.1 Using metaphors

Using metaphors or visual images to remember and describe symptoms is a good technique for jogging your memory. It can be an effective way to communicate degrees of physical, mental, or emotional pain. Look at the following examples:

- "It feels like my shoulder has been pierced by an arrow."

- "My stomach feels bruised."

- "My muscles feel as if they are on fire."

- Someone describing loneliness might say, "My heart feels overwhelmed with grief."

- A phrase such as "I feel as though I'm carrying a heavy knapsack on my back" can describe an overwhelming sense of responsibility.

There are many words or images you can choose to describe your pain or ailment. The point is to find an accurate expression or picture to describe exactly how you feel.

For example, after an accident while playing hockey, John felt as if his knee would explode. He was able to draw on his imagination and his experience with a similar injury along with the physical signs of injury to help his doctor understand what was wrong.

"I can see that you are in a lot of pain," said the doctor. "Where does it hurt most?"

"Here," said John, pointing to the side of his knee. "This is where it hurts."

The doctor gently touched the knee. "It's quite swollen," he said.

"It's burning ... throbbing," said John, groaning. "Give me something, please, to ease the pain."

"First tell me how deep the pain is," said the doctor. "Can you describe it?"

"It feels as if a knife is piercing a nerve."

"I see," said the doctor. "Has it been gradual?"

"Yes, it started slowly," said John. "But then it suddenly got worse."

By describing his pain as burning, throbbing, and piercing, John gave his doctor an exact picture of the depth of his pain. The doctor could quickly assess the degree of discomfort for John, which allowed for speedier treatment and recovery.

1.2 Using humor

Humor can be helpful in some circumstances, leaving the patient and doctor more relaxed; however, mismatched styles of humor will result in a flat response. If the humor styles match, more than likely you will both enjoy a chuckle.

Humor can also ease an awkward or embarrassing moment between the patient and the doctor. The effect will depend on whether both people share a similar sense of humor. Some people might not appreciate certain types of humor, such as dry, flippant, or dark humor; other people might respond better to visual or risky humor, or to light humor, or even to somewhat risqué humor. Tongue-in-cheek or dry humor can be very useful for deflecting awkward situations.

Louise, an infrequent visitor to her primary physician, made an appointment for an annual physical. As a busy executive in a large corporation she felt very much in control of her life. Yet, she felt tense about the upcoming internal exam before arriving at the doctor's office, even though she had been seeing this doctor for several years.

Once in the examining room, Louise undressed and put the gown on that the doctor had left for her. When the doctor returned, he asked her a few questions about how she was feeling, checked her respiratory functions and her heart and blood flow. He listened to her responses to his questions and then asked her to lie back on the examining table. Then he examined her breasts and abdomen.

Just as the doctor began the pelvic exam, a cell phone rang. Both the doctor and Louise, embarrassed, looked around to identify whose cell had beeped. Immediately they looked at the other, realized the absurdity of the situation, and burst out laughing. Then Louise blurted out, "I guess my happy spot set off some bells!" The comment was so spontaneous that it threw them both off. However, the awkwardness of the situation caused both the doctor and patient to laugh even more. The tension in this situation certainly was decreased, which in turn created a more relaxed interaction between both individuals.

In this particular case, Louise's reaction was quick-witted and confident and lightened the situation. It helped that she and the doctor were familiar with one another, so her wit did not offend him. (By the way, it's usually a good idea to turn off your cell phone before you go into the doctor's office!)

Doctors, too, are quite familiar with this type of humor, especially when trying to diffuse the effect of a frustrating or unhappy medical case. Often remarks along these lines are spontaneous. A patient may respond in a similar manner, particularly if he or she has been given a negative medical prognosis. It not only diffuses the effect of the news, but also delays the final emotional impact.

Although humor can help in some situations, there are a few things to keep in mind before using this approach. Because one person's sense of humor might differ from another's, there is a risk of causing offense. You might laugh at one thing and someone else might frown. Humor certainly helps in a variety of situations, but there are those moments when other communication strategies are better.

1.3 Communicating with an aloof doctor

When you communicate, you use your voice and your body to express what you feel and want, or don't feel and don't want. Your tone of voice and its inflection, whether or not you make eye contact, and your body language play a role in how your message is received.

The same is true for the doctor. If the doctor doesn't look you in the eye, or sits in a slouched position, or perhaps always stands tall with arms crossed, your impression might be of a doctor who is defensive or arrogant. You might, without realizing, mirror the doctor's communication style. Such an atmosphere will likely be uncomfortable for both of you and misunderstandings can occur. How can you respond when your doctor appears aloof? Consider the following scenario:

Omar usually visits his GP once a year, but he has made two or three visits in the last month with the same complaint — migraines. His marriage recently broke up and his work situation is suffering. The headaches have increased in the last several months.

Neither Omar nor the doctor has discussed any possible reason for the migraines other than a chemical imbalance. His doctor appears indifferent. Omar's third visit went like this:

Omar was waiting in the doctor's office when the doctor walked in, reading his file as she went over to her desk and sat down. She glanced up at him and asked, "What is the problem today?"

"These headaches are getting worse," said Omar. "I can't sleep, and I can't get any work done. They just hurt so much I can hardly stand it."

"Hmmm," said the doctor, leaning back in her chair. Her tone remained cool and matter-of-fact. "What have you taken for the pain?"

"I've tried a variety of the painkillers I could find on the shelf at the drugstore. But nothing works. I need something stronger."

"Here, try this." She scribbled something on a prescription pad. "It should help relieve the headache." She stood up to hand Omar the piece of paper and then went over to the door. "That's all for today, right?"

"Well, uh," said Omar, taken by surprise. "Shouldn't I come for a follow-up?"

"Call the receptionist if you think you need to. Otherwise, I'll see you when you come in for your annual checkup."

Omar never expected such a cool response from his doctor. He felt as if she was not interested in him at all; in fact, he felt ignored. How could he take control of the situation, to make sure he gets the care he needs? One possibility is to get angry and demand more time from the doctor. Or he could have left without saying anything and gone to his local community clinic, where he might have received a warmer reception. He could also have chosen to confront his doctor to tell her directly how he felt about their interaction. Let's see what might have happened if he had provided more information about his symptoms at the beginning of his visit. Let's rewind and start over:

When the doctor came into the office reading Omar's medical file, Omar waited until she was finished before he started talking. When she looked up, he said, "Doctor, my headaches have become a lot worse since my wife and I separated last month. They're interfering with my work, and I'm finding it difficult to concentrate. I've tried taking over-the-counter painkillers, like you suggested last time, but they don't seem very effective. I don't know what to do."

Omar has taken the position of knowing something about his situation and how it may be contributing to his symptoms. He is providing the doctor with meaningful background information.

"Oh," said the doctor, "I didn't know about all these changes in your life. They could certainly be increasing your tension levels. That could be a reason for your headaches." Her voice sounds calm and sympathetic. "How about if I check a few other things?"

"Okay," responds Omar. Her manner relaxes him and he starts to feel as though together they will be able to find the cause and the solution to his migraines.

As she checks his blood pressure, she asks Omar to tell her more about what's going on in his life. "Let's just chat now for a few minutes, and then you can come back next week and we can discuss ways to help you get through this tough period in your life."

"Sure," says Omar. "That sounds good." He finds it easy to open up to her and tell her how he feels about the breakup of his marriage and the stresses of his job. By the end of the 15-minute visit he already feels more relaxed.

Granted, this is an ideal scenario, but often a broad opening statement with lots of information can lead to a more productive exchange between you and the doctor. By speaking up, you are taking a more assertive stance with your health communication, even though it is the doctor's larger responsibility to inquire about symptoms, especially by the second visit.

2. What Your Doctor Should Know

Often we don't let the doctor know of the upsets, stresses, and minor injuries in our personal lives, even though they might contribute to changes in our mental or physical health. For example, these apparently small details can aggravate conditions such as depression, migraines, backaches, fatigue, and stomach pain.

2.1 Family medical history

Similarly, we often forget to inform the doctor of crucial family history that might affect diagnosis, prognosis, intervention, and even short- or long-term medical treatment. A family's medical past might include many conditions with hereditary factors, such as heart disease, stroke, mental illness, or certain types of cancer. If you and your doctor know about these patterns, you can discuss what symptoms to watch for and what preventive measures to take.

For example, on Paula's mother's side of the family there is a history of stroke. When Paula's grandfather had a stroke, she began to learn more about the condition. She became concerned about her own risk of stroke, so she booked an appointment with her doctor to discuss it.

"It never occurred to me to tell you about the history of strokes in my family," Paula told her doctor. "I had no idea that it existed until my mother's father's stroke last year. My mother told me that her grandfather had died of a stroke, too."

"I see," said the doctor, taking notes. "I'm glad you're telling me now. Better late than never!"

"Then a friend told me that chronic stress can add to the risk of stroke," Paula said. "I have a high-stress job, you know, and right now it's a tough time for me; my stress levels are even higher than usual. So I began to worry."

"I think it's premature to start worrying, Paula," said the doctor. "A family history of stroke is no guarantee that you'll have one too, and there are lots of things you can do to reduce the risk." She explained some of the things Paula could do to cut down her risk of stroke. She finished up by saying, "You were right to tell me about this possibility. It gives me a good reference for making sure you get the right medical care, and means we can work together to keep you as healthy as possible."

Paula left the doctor's office feeling very relieved — plus she went home with a lot of accurate information about strokes.

2.2 Communicating discomfort

You should inform your doctor if you feel uncomfortable with any aspect of your routine annual checkup. For example, it's important to tell your doctor if you're uneasy with groin or rectal examinations or breast examinations. Your doctor will try to interact with you in a way that decreases your discomfort or nervousness. If you still do not feel comfortable, you might consider finding another doctor. If you do, be sure to inform the new doctor of your concerns. The problem may not be the doctor, but your own aversion to invasive procedures.

For example, Roger couldn't get used to having his doctor examine his lower body for any reason.

"At first, I thought it might be my doctor and his style of interaction," he told his friend, Larry.

"I hate those examinations!" said Larry. "So what did you do — go to another doctor?"

"Not just one! I went to several," Roger said with a laugh. "Eventually I figured out that it had more to do with me than with the doctors."

"What did you do?"

"I was actually relieved to go back to my original doctor because I'd known him since I was a kid. I explained what had happened, and he seemed to understand."

"Weren't you still uncomfortable?"

"Well, yes," said Roger. "But he was pretty good about listening to me. During the exam he distracted me so I ended up not getting so tense."

"I can't imagine what would distract me enough ... how'd he do it?"

"It was kind of funny, actually," said Roger. "He just asked me a couple of questions about my kids and then we started talking about sailing, and before I knew it the whole thing was over."

"Gee," said Larry. "You've given me some ideas for my next checkup!"

Men and women frequently feel uncomfortable or embarrassed about such procedures. Some people manage to think about other things during the exam, but some people can't help themselves from cringing or wincing. The doctor can help make it easier. Discussing your concerns will usually bring about an understanding response, and the exam won't be so unpleasant.

2.3 Discussing physical symptoms

It's important to tell your doctor about changes in your body, such as unusual lumps, rashes, or persistent pain. That gives your doctor the opportunity to discuss any worries or concerns you might have, and also allows for early detection of possibly serious conditions.

Byron, for example, had unbearably itchy feet and ankles, but his feet were so smelly he was too embarrassed even to let his doctor near them. He became so worried that his condition was incurable that it began to influence his daily functioning. He went to great lengths to disguise the problem at work and with friends. He dredged his socks in baby powder to decrease the odor while at work or in social situations and kept his shoes on whenever possible. This behavior only inflamed the rash and increased the itchiness, particularly during the night.

His rampant thoughts about imaginary diseases with devastating results began to consume him. Byron finally had no choice but to visit his doctor. Before departing for the doctor's office he again filled his socks with baby powder. Once there, he stammered and hesitated, and eventually blurted out the problem. He told his doctor that he was so anxious about his feet that he imagined he had some awful condition like that flesh-eating disease that was in the news a few years ago. He was convinced that even his doctor wouldn't be able to stand the smell and sight of his feet, but she persuaded him to take off his shoes and socks and diagnosed a simple case of athlete's foot. She prescribed a treatment plan that gave Byron immediate relief.

2.4 Communicating about emotional symptoms

Just as it's useful for the doctor to know about the family medical history, it's also helpful to let the doctor know about the family's behavioral and emotional coping skills that might relate to family tensions. This history might relate to your own coping skills. This kind of information is particularly important if you find yourself thinking about or re-enacting some kind of destructive behavior as a response to life stresses.

For example, when he was between 10 and 15 years old, Tony regularly heard his father raging about the family's financial difficulty. His father's behavior led to intense arguing and verbal abuse toward Tony's mother and other members of the family.

When Tony was 30, he experienced similar frustration when he was laid off. Fortunately he felt comfortable talking with his doctor about the possibility of repeating the behavior he had observed in his father.

"I didn't start to worry about my behavior until a few weeks after I lost my job," he told his sister, Margaret. "I began feeling resentful toward the company, and then one day I just blew up before breakfast."

"In front of Susie and the kids?"

"Yes, it was awful," said Tony. "The anger welled up so quickly that I just swept everything off the table. The look of horror on Jamie and Annie's faces … and Susie looked so afraid … it jolted me right back to reality."

"Ooh, that sounds familiar," said Margaret.

"I know," said Tony. "It was just like the way Dad used to behave."

"What did you do?" asked Margaret. "You seem to be much more relaxed now."

"You know how destructive Dad's behavior was. As soon as I realized I was repeating it, I talked to Susie about it, and she suggested I see the doctor," said Tony. "So I did. And you know what? He didn't judge me or make me feel guilty at all! In fact, I told him about Dad and he listened, and now I'm seeing him once a week until I get through this."

"Is this your GP you're talking about?" asked Margaret.

"Yes, it is. He offered to refer me to a psychologist or a counselor if I'd rather see someone else," Tony said. "But I was comfortable talking to him, and he seems skilled enough."

"That's great," said Margaret. "Sounds like you're handling the situation well."

2.5 Mental disorders and feeling alone

Certain mental illness disorders, such as Alzheimer's disease or other forms of dementia, present their own challenges. In many cases, relatives and friends have to look after the needs of the patients, but someone with no family or close friends has another dimension of aloneness, fear, and challenges. That person must depend on the doctor's arrangements or make formal arrangements for care in the early stages of the condition.

Matthew's doctor told him that he was in the early stages of Alzheimer's. At 59, he was widowed with no children and living alone. Matthew was very frightened. His personal support system was basically nonexistent. He began to shake when his doctor gave him the news. He asked the doctor what he should do. Who would help him? How long would it be before the disease would interfere with his everyday functions? Why did the disease strike him and not someone else? His doctor answered as many questions as he could, and arranged for Matthew to meet with a specialist and a support counselor from the Alzheimer Society. Mathew was able to attend information sessions and receive counseling through the society. He was also guided toward nursing homes that provided long-term care for people with Alzheimer's. That he was still able to search and make decisions about his care and living situation gave him a sense of control over his future. He began to feel somewhat assured that as his condition worsened there would be a guardian in place as well as a long-term facility with a good health-care team that would care for him.

2.6 Lifestyle challenges

You may want to discuss with your doctor any concerns associated with stressful living conditions, multiple sex partners, sleep disturbances, persistent emotional upset, or just the frustrations you feel from dealing with life's challenges.

Jennie, for example, had unprotected sex with about 25 sex partners over ten years. When she was 35, she became engaged and hoped to have children. Her whole lifestyle and outlook changed. Aware that her past behavior put her and others at risk, she thought she should have herself checked for sexually transmitted diseases. However, she hesitated to tell the doctor the truth about her previous risky lifestyle. She knew it was in the past, but she didn't want to share that part of her life with anyone. Plus she was afraid of what she might find out, and she was afraid that the doctor might make her feel guilty. She knew that if she withheld the information from her doctor, she might end up passing something on to her current partner, and she didn't want to take that risk. Her only responsible choice was to talk to her doctor. To her surprise, the doctor not only understood but even praised Jennie for telling him. When the doctor tested her for sexually transmitted diseases, Jennie fortunately tested negative; she was disease free.

2.7 Life support choices

Telling the doctor about personal circumstances, past, and present behavior is important, just as is talking about any recurring or worrisome ailments. Some people also consider it important to discuss with their doctor how they would like to be treated medically and personally if they are ever incapacitated.

Joelle felt very strongly that she should never be placed on life support if her health deteriorated to a life-threatening level. She had drawn up a document for medical power of attorney (also known as a living will or health-care directive) and included an amendment that specified her wishes. She had a notarized letter explaining her wishes placed in her medical file as a reference.

Derek informed his doctor that he did not want his cancer to be treated aggressively with various medicines or medical technologies. His research told him that there was little chance of survival despite treatment. He did not want to prolong his life and he didn't want to be in pain. His only preference was to receive pain medication to enable him to die as free of pain as possible.

Tyler had been told that he had untreatable complications from AIDS. He wanted to use marijuana as a treatment for pain. This situation presented a problem for the doctor, who wanted to assist Tyler with reducing his pain but at the same time did not want to support the use of marijuana. Because the treatment plan still presented legal problems in most of North America, his doctor could not support his choice. However, the doctor did sympathize and recommended that Tyler talk with a herbalist informed about other forms of legal herbal pain management substances. Tyler understood and appreciated the doctor's suggestions and moral support.

Many facets of ourselves contribute to how we communicate with the doctor: moods, style, perception, willingness to listen, attention span, humor, choices, and so on. Skill is a large part of successfully and effectively getting our point across. Effort is significant, for without effort, skill has no chance to develop. Our purpose is to practice our communication skills, and to work toward taking a greater interest in wellness.

3. The Challenge of Remembering

Remembering can be a challenge, especially with the multitude of activities in our daily lives, from attending to children, maintaining personal and working relationships, and trying to keep up with the cost of living. It seems a lot to ask of someone to remember to make an annual appointment with the doctor, let alone arrive fully prepared to brief the doctor.

Forgetting what we want to say can stem from preoccupation, stress, nervousness, disinterest, or persistent pain, not to mention how much time passes between appointments. Some people think seeing the doctor every few years is sufficient. A few people feel no need to see a doctor at all. However, many of us see the doctor on an annual basis, and most of us see the doctor several times a year. Remembering what we want to say is a skill that requires concentration and effort.

3.1 Forgetting the reason for your visit

Have you ever heard someone say, "I went to see my doctor and forgot to tell her about ... ?" Or, "I arrived at the doctor's office and drew a blank about the nature of my complaint." It happens all the time. Sometime between the time you leave for the doctor's appointment and the time you arrive in the waiting room and the moment you enter the examining room you forget your purpose in seeing the doctor. You might remember some of the complaints, but forget the rest. Or sometimes you remember what it is you wanted to discuss, but you leave the office without remembering any of the advice your doctor gave you.

For example, Chris arrived at his appointment on time, but waited 45 minutes before seeing his doctor. In the examining room, the doctor said, "My medical clerk tells me that you reported having headaches, constipation, tiredness, and strained vision in the last few days. How are you feeling now?"

"Fine," said Chris.

If Chris feels fine, then why did he make an appointment to see his doctor? Maybe in the time lag between booking the appointment and seeing the doctor he had forgotten what made him book the appointment in the first place. Or, perhaps, in the presence of the doctor he felt awkward, so he drew a blank on the reason for his visit. In fact, Chris visits his doctor frequently and more often than not he forgets the exact reason for the visit, so this time he made a list of his symptoms to assist his memory.

The list stated: headache, tiredness, constipation, and strained vision.

Chris could expand on these points by indicating the intensity of discomfort he was experiencing as well as how long he'd been feeling them. For example, he could jot down specific symptoms associated with his main complaint:

- Headaches: pounding, gripping (from front to back of skull) — three days.

- Constipation: feeling bulky, bloated, no bowel movement — four days.

- Tiredness: general malaise, sluggishness, lasts all day — one week.

- Strained vision: slight blurring, sore dry eyes — three days.

This gave Chris's doctor a clear outline of his condition.

3.2 Forgetting to visit the doctor

In contrast, Chris's wife, Natasha, often completely forgets to visit the doctor for her annual checkup. In fact, visiting the doctor is the least of her priorities.

"I am very busy and healthy," she said to Chris. "If not for you, I'd easily not even think about seeing the doctor for years."

"But you know, honey, I keep reading that women should see their doctors at least every year."

"We have this conversation every year!" said Natasha, laughing. "It's the only way I remember to book an appointment."

There are a few things Natasha could do to remind herself to call her doctor's office for an appointment instead of relying solely on Chris:

- She could make a follow-up appointment while she's at the doctor's office.

- She could ask the doctor's medical office assistant to give her a reminder call.

- She could enter the date in red ink in her agenda book, program it into her cell phone reminders app, or add it to her calendar.

- She could book the appointment close to her birthday and make it a habit to do so every year.

- She could set aside two hours on the day of the appointment to include travel time to and from the doctor's office as well as the waiting time and the actual appointment.

When Natasha does see the doctor, she should be specific about asking the doctor for suggestions to continue her good health. Once at home, she should write down the doctor's suggestions and read any pamphlets given to her.

3.3 Forgetting how to describe the pain

Physical or emotional discomfort can hinder the quality of what we remember. A young child, for instance, will remember a nicked finger because the pain is something new or is a major event. An adult might ignore the same discomfort and describe it as nothing. The memory of the discomfort for one is sustained longer than for the other.

Someone with a persistent ache may be more inclined to have a description of the pain that is concise. Or the symptoms might be multiple and difficult to describe. Others experience pain routinely, perhaps because of the nature of their work or activities, so they learn to suppress the pain temporarily. But because the pain that sends them to the doctor is so intense, they may have difficulty retrieving words to describe it.

For example, Mario has a pain in his hip incurred from an old sports injury. As a result, he has trained himself to minimize the pain. Over time, he has developed visualization techniques to change how he perceives it.

When Mario played amateur soccer, it was not unusual for him to push the pain aside in his mind, so he could continue to play. In some ways, the game was more important than taking care of the pain. Distorting his perception of it led to his inability to describe the pain adequately. Mario could find various ways to describe the pain to his doctor:

- Remember when and how the pain started.

- Remember words that best describe the ache or pain.

- Remember what makes the pain worse.

- Remember what makes the pain lessen.

- Write a list of the actual aches, pains, or injuries, which he could show to the doctor.

By thinking ahead about your symptoms and the reason for your visit, you are in a better position to remember and describe your symptoms to the doctor. A concise and clearly written list, with a description of the purpose of your visit, will save you and the doctor a lot of time.

4. When You and Your Doctor Disagree

Most of us have disagreed on occasion with our doctor's approach or treatment recommendations. We might not have openly expressed our thoughts at the time or at all. As a result, we might feel annoyed, resentful, or indifferent toward the doctor. Because of such feelings, we might avoid going to the doctor or tune out during a visit. Eventually the confidence and respect we might have had for the doctor begins to dwindle. The relationship has deteriorated partly because of the reluctance to negotiate differences of opinion. With the absence of negotiation, there is no opportunity to have our views heard. The dynamic, then, is that the relationship is one-sided, leaving us feeling as though there's no point in saying anything. However, it doesn't have to be this way.

4.1 Making sure you are heard

As in any relationship, part of negotiating differences of opinion is being willing to listen to one another. If you do not feel you are heard, then you might feel there is little possibility for successful negotiation. In such instances, you might just have to walk away.

For example, Micheline, a former nurse, reported to her GP that she had lower back pain as well as abdominal cramping overnight. He examined her, suggested that she might have an intestinal condition called Crohn's disease, and scheduled some tests with a specialist. Micheline had a history of stomach trouble, which she had diagnosed herself as irritable bowel syndrome, and that history combined with her medical knowledge led her to think her pain was related in some way to a kidney problem. Her GP and the specialist disagreed with her. Even with her knowledge, she didn't feel strong enough to negotiate with either of them, so she went along with the tests.

One of the tests required Micheline to stay in the hospital for a day. While she was resting after the test, the specialist told Micheline she had irritable bowel syndrome. When she told the specialist that she had already figured that out on her own he didn't even acknowledge that she had been right. When she told him her left side, near her kidneys, still felt uncomfortable, he dismissed it as an after-effect of the test. Micheline was still groggy from the anesthetic used in the test, and didn't feel up to arguing with him. When he patted her on the knee and said he would check back again shortly, she felt completely ignored and angry.

When the doctor returned, the anesthetic had almost completely worn off. This time Micheline was more assertive, and drew on her knowledge of her own medical history as well as her medical background.

"How are you feeling now?" asked the doctor.

"The anesthetic has almost worn off," she replied. "I continue to have pain, though. I think I should have an ultrasound to see if the problem is in my kidney area."

"Well, my dear," said the doctor, a little taken aback. "I know that's what you feel, but I really don't think … "

"Doctor, I know what you think," said Micheline, clearly annoyed. "I know this pain is still persistent and I insist that an ultrasound be done." Her voice was firm. "Otherwise, I will have to file a complaint."

"All right, all right," said the doctor. "You'll have the test as soon as possible." Without another word, he turned and headed to the nursing station to make the arrangements.

Micheline's sense of frustration and annoyance that neither of her doctors were willing to listen left her very upset. What could Micheline have done differently?

There are many ways to make sure your opinions are heard:

- Describe the place and quality of the pain as accurately as possible.

- Take a stronger stand with your GP before having further procedures.

- Ask a friend or relative to accompany you for support in negotiating your needs.

- Seek a second opinion before agreeing to a procedure.

In the end, Micheline decided to look for another GP who was more willing to listen to her and negotiate alternative methods of diagnosing her condition. She knew she would not have to interact with the specialist again.

4.2 Negotiating differences of opinions

When two people negotiate differences of opinion there must be a common goal of mutual gain. There must also be a willingness to listen to one another's views as well as to compromise on some issues. If you keep an open mind and respect your own convictions, you and your doctor can reach a consensus on final decisions about your health care.

Liza had her first child, Haley, when she was in her mid-40s. She had read a lot on homeopathic health care for infants, including the pros and cons of giving vaccinations to children. She had read that vaccinating a child can be hazardous for a child's long-term health. Liza's doctor was inclined to follow the conventional practices of preventive care. When Liza took Haley in for her regular checkup, everything went smoothly until the doctor suggested it was time for Haley to have her first vaccinations.

"No way," said Liza. "Vaccinations are dangerous. I don't want to expose Haley to the risks of conventional vaccinations."

"What do you mean by risks?" asked the doctor. "Vaccinations are a protection against certain diseases."

"I've heard that some vaccinations can have a bad effect on the immune system," said Liza, shaking her head. "I don't want to put my baby at risk."

"Where did you hear such a thing?"

Liza recognized a derogatory tone in the doctor's voice. "I read an article in a local magazine on homeopathic treatments," she replied defensively.

"Listen, Liza," said the doctor, "loving parents give their children vaccinations."

"Are you suggesting that I do not love my child because I won't subject her to vaccinations?" Liza asked angrily.

"Well, no." Now it was the doctor's turn to sound defensive. "But I know you would want to do the best for your child."

"As a matter of fact I do and that is why I have chosen a more natural route. I will have to find someone else who has a similar outlook to mine." She took Haley and left the doctor's office, determined to find another doctor.

Liza and her doctor arrived at a single solution, which was to terminate the relationship; however, neither one of them examined alternative solutions that could have resulted in mutual gain. What could Liza have done to take better control of the situation? Once it was clear to her that the doctor did not share her view, she could have directed the conversation differently. Their conversation could have gone like this:

"I understand your concern," said Liza , when the doctor suggested vaccinating Haley. "But I've recently read that vaccinations can actually have a negative effect on my baby's immune system."

"Oh?" said the doctor. "Where did you read that?"

"In a magazine article. It quoted some case studies of children having severe reactions to the vaccination. Some even developed some of the diseases they were being vaccinated against."

"I can give you other information on the benefits of vaccines for children. Take a look at this pamphlet, for starters," said the doctor, as she took a brochure from his desk drawer. "Do you have a copy of that article you read? I'd like to read it."

"It so happens I do!" Liza said with a smile. "I brought it just in case you asked me about it."

"Great," said the doctor. "How about you read up on the arguments for immunization, and I'll read up on the arguments against, and we meet again in a week to discuss our findings."

"Sure," replied Liza. "I'll see you then. Thanks!"

Obviously, this approach produced a more favorable outcome. Liza was able to explain her views and the doctor respected her opinion. Liza can consider the doctor's information and still remain with her own views, and likewise the doctor may remain with his position. Perhaps they will agree to a balance of choices. Either way, Liza and her doctor made an effort to explore options that could lead to an amicable solution.

4.3 Negotiating your position

On occasion there can be discrepancies between information reported in a medical file and verbal reports on your health condition. Because the accuracy of such information is important, this is something that without question needs pursuing until it is corrected. You might have to be persistent, but you must firmly insist that corrections are made before you can negotiate any treatment. You need strong motivation, especially if your doctor appears reluctant to act.

In Ruth's case, her GP referred her to a specialist for treatment for an acidic stomach. The specialist told Ruth she did not have an ulcer. The GP, however, told Ruth that the written report indicated positive findings of an ulcer. Ruth told her doctor she was confused by the different reports.

"The report from the specialist says you have an ulcer," repeated the doctor, as he wrote out a prescription. "This medication has shown great results ... "

"The specialist told me that he found nothing wrong," said Ruth. "He said everything was okay. I don't understand." The doctor looked at the report again.

"It's written here that indications of an ulcer were found."

"Can I please see the report?" asked Ruth. The doctor handed it to her, and she could see that it stated clearly "ulcers were found."

"This doesn't make any sense," said Ruth. "I don't understand. The specialist distinctly said there was nothing wrong."

"I'm sorry, Ruth, but I can only go by what the report says."

"I don't want to take any drugs until I know for certain what's going on," said Ruth.

"Perhaps you should check with the specialist," the GP suggested.

Disappointed, Ruth left the doctor's office. She telephoned the specialist, who assured her that the results of her tests were negative. Ruth called her GP back and repeated this information. In response, the GP asked Ruth to have the specialist fax another copy of the report to the GP.

"This is so frustrating!" said Ruth, exasperated. "Why should I be the one trying to straighten out what it says in the actual report? I mean, I understand that you are busy," she continued, in calmer tone of voice. "But I really think you ought to call the specialist yourself. Then we can discuss the real findings. Shall I book an appointment for the day after tomorrow? Meanwhile, what can I do to help my stomach feel better?"

Ruth's first reaction was an angry one, but she realized that to make progress she needed to get some things out in the open. She plainly said that she didn't like being the go-between between her doctor and the specialist. By empathizing with the GP about his busy schedule, Ruth did not antagonize the doctor, and she clarified what she expected the doctor's role to be. Plus she kept control of the situation by suggesting a time line. Her doctor quickly recognized that Ruth was taking an active role in her treatment.

"You're right," said the doctor. "I'll call the specialist and talk to him directly."

"Thank you." Ruth was relieved that the doctor was willing to negotiate on her behalf.

"Stick with a bland diet for the next couple of days," the doctor continued. "Try to avoid acidic foods for now. If you can drop by the office later, I can give you a list of foods to avoid."

"Okay, I think I can get there this afternoon. Shall I make an appointment while I'm at it?"

"Let me talk to the specialist first," said the doctor. "Then I'll call you in a few days."

"Thank you," said Ruth. "Could you let me know if you don't hear back from the specialist within two days?" She was grateful for the doctor's efforts on her behalf, but she wanted to make sure the doctor understood she wasn't willing to wait too long.

"Yes," answered the doctor. "Either I'll call you myself or I'll have the medical clerk call."

Satisfied, Ruth was able to take some steps to make herself more comfortable while she waited for the doctor and the specialist to discuss the report. Despite her early frustration, she firmly stood her ground, agreeing to negotiate possible treatment only once the discrepancy in the medical report was clarified. When the GP and the specialist reviewed the written report, they found it contained a mistake: The specialist had written "found" instead of "not found" and the GP called Ruth to discuss the appropriate treatment plan.

A higher percentage of women today are reaching the menopausal stage of their lives. Many in this age group have firm convictions about hormone replacement therapy (HRT) and its possible side effects. Women also have more choices in dealing with the various stages of menopause. Because of the availability of information on various conventional medicines and herbal treatments for menopause, women are now in a stronger position to negotiate and decide their treatment preferences.

Julia is 48 years old and experiences night sweats, irritability, weight gain, and fatigue. She feels miserable. To complicate matters, there is a history of heart disease and breast cancer in her family. Because of these factors, she wanted to discuss her fears with her doctor.

"I've really read a lot about the benefits and risks of HRT," Julia told her doctor. "Given my history I am not comfortable with this option, but I do want to do something because these symptoms are really driving me crazy!"

"What other options are you interested in trying?" asked her doctor.

"I'm intrigued by the idea of natural supplements. I read that supplements such as vitamin E and the B vitamins, can help, and I've heard a lot about evening primrose oil. Several things I've read recommend exercise and reducing the amount of animal fat in my diet. I'm not sure if any of this will work. In some ways, I'd like a quick fix."

"I'm sorry I have no miracle cures," said the doctor with a smile. "I think that the conventional approach is usually best, but I'm willing to try something else. Have you tried anything on your own?"

"I've started experimenting with taking vitamins and keeping track of my diet, and I started exercising a bit," said Julia, "but that's only been for a week. It seems like a good way to go, but how much do you know about this approach?"

"I'm not an expert," said the doctor, "but it's certainly becoming a popular approach. I think we both need to know a bit more about it."

"I have an article at home I could bring you, if you like."

"Sure, I'd be happy to look at it when I get a chance," said the doctor. "Let's set a follow-up appointment in about four weeks to further explore your options."

Julia and her doctor reached a tentative solution in their negotiation. Both were receptive to listening to the other and open to exploring alternatives in reaching a possible consensus on treatment. Fortunately Julia had the option of negotiating with her doctor about treatment. Not every patient has this luxury or opportunity, especially if the doctor is an unwilling participant.

You are in a better position to negotiate or communicate what you want if you are informed and capable of choosing one treatment over another. If, in this instance, the GP is not willing to consider options, then you can request an opinion from another doctor more willing to look at alternatives. Keep in mind that if you do not agree with a doctor's diagnosis, prognosis, or prescribed treatment, it does not label you as an uncooperative or difficult patient. Rather, it presents you as a responsible, intelligent, and willing participant in addressing your health-care needs.

5. When You Are Dissatisfied or Satisfied

Expressing how you feel to the doctor is important. However, not everyone is open to hearing your dissatisfaction, especially if that person is the target of your criticism. Choosing the right time is important, as is figuring out how to make your point without causing offense. Diplomatic tactics at such times are preferable, provided you do not sacrifice your viewpoint. That old adage that honey is sweeter than vinegar is often true, as long as sincerity is a critical ingredient.

5.1 Feeling ignored and dissatisfied

Zoe's story is a good example of how to let a doctor know that something is wrong. During her first year of graduate studies, she began to experience unusual vaginal bleeding. A few years earlier, a routine Pap smear had revealed a condition that could have led to cervical cancer. That had been treated successfully, but this time she thought it was best to see a doctor as soon as possible.

Her university was four hours away from her hometown so she had to travel a distance for an appointment made for the following week. When Zoe arrived for her appointment at 10:30 in the morning there was no one in the office. She waited for about 20 minutes before the medical office assistant arrived. The doctor arrived in the office another 20 minutes later. Zoe thought it wouldn't be much longer until she saw the doctor, but another 20 minutes passed. By now, an hour after the appointed time, Zoe was anxious. She had a four-hour drive back to the university for an evening class she did not want to miss. It was close to noon when she was finally called into the doctor's office.

"I think I'd better come back another time," said Zoe. "I have to get back to the university now."

The doctor looked at Zoe's file. "Considering your symptoms, I think you should have an exam."

Zoe looked at her watch. The doctor said, "Your symptoms sound to me like a possibility of cervical cancer; you should be examined, now."

Zoe was not happy with this situation. She felt awkward with her doctor, and the combination of the possible seriousness of her condition and the lack of time made her tense. She felt she had no choice.

"All right," she said. "I guess I'll be late for evening class."

To her relief, the results of Zoe's examination showed no sign of the earlier condition. Even though the threat of cancer was gone, she was still dissatisfied with the way she had been treated at the doctor's. For weeks afterward she was upset. Both the doctor and her medical office assistant took Zoe's time for granted. Zoe felt the doctor's attitude was arrogant and intimidating, and her assumption that Zoe might have cancer, without even having examined her, was especially disturbing. Zoe thought the doctor was very irresponsible in her communication. She decided to discuss her feelings with the doctor.

Zoe made long-distance telephone calls to the doctor several times without success. Either the line was busy or the answering service picked up. Her calls were never returned. Finally, she wrote a letter to the doctor explaining that she would like to discuss her last visit. She asked the doctor to reply either by telephone or letter. She received no response.

Just as she had felt she had no option when she was in the doctor's office, Zoe felt she had no choice but to go over the doctor's head. She decided that the only way to receive any satisfaction was to send another letter to the GP explaining her complaint, with a copy to the medical complaints committee of the Royal College of Physicians and Surgeons. As a result, the College investigated the matter and Zoe received a written and verbal apology from the doctor. The doctor's explanation was that she did not make long-distance phone calls and time did not permit her to write a letter.

Although she didn't fully understand the reason behind the doctor's behavior, Zoe was glad to get some form of apology. However, she didn't see why she should have to go to such lengths to be treated courteously.

5.2 Feeling disrespected

When we visit the doctor we expect that our privacy will be respected. We also expect that the doctor will speak to us in a respectful manner.

After two years, Tommy made an appointment for a regular checkup. When the doctor walked into the examining room, he took one look at Tommy's chart and one look at Tommy and said, "I see last time you were here, you weighed about 31 pounds less than you do now. Looks like you've been doing a little overeating since then?"

Tommy was dumbfounded by the doctor's blunt comments; he said nothing.

"Tommy, how about we do a complete physical today. Put this on and I'll be back in a moment." The doctor handed Tommy a gown and stepped out of the office.

As Tommy was undressing, the door opened and the doctor's assistant walked in. Tommy quickly covered himself up. She glanced at him, put a document on the doctor's desk and without a word, left. Tommy finished putting on the gown and sat down in the chair to wait.

A moment later, the doctor returned. "Get up on the table," he said curtly.

As Tommy stepped onto the stool to climb on to the examining table, his foot slipped and he fell to the floor. The doctor made no effort to help Tommy get up. Tommy felt humiliated. Everything was becoming more and more uncomfortable. Finally, he spoke up.

"Doctor, I don't feel comfortable having you do the exam," he said.

"It's your choice," said the doctor with a shrug. "What's the problem?"

"You made a negative comment about my weight when you first entered this room. Then your assistant barged into the room while I was changing; she didn't even apologize! Then you order me over to the table, and just now ... " Tommy was starting to get angry. "You didn't even bother to help me when I slipped. I think I'd rather have a doctor who's respectful and professional, who treats me like a human!"

"I'm sorry ... I didn't realize ... " The doctor seemed taken aback. "Would you like a referral to someone else?"

"Not a chance! I prefer to find another doctor myself," said Tommy. "Now, would you please leave the room while I change back into my clothes?" If Tommy is serious about finding a new doctor, he might first have to go to a walk-in clinic.

Although Tommy had been unduly humiliated and treated with disrespect, he remained calm when he expressed his dissatisfaction with the doctor. He stuck to the facts. He used an assertive and firm tone, and left no room for the doctor to argue with him. Tommy took a stand by first stating how he felt and describing the situation and then explaining to the doctor the consequences of the behavior.

5.3 Feeling rushed

The doctor's medical clerk or receptionist often sets the tone for your visit with the doctor. This is one reason why you need to be clear with the receptionist about your reasons for wanting to see the doctor. If you do not, you might feel rushed because of the doctor's tight schedule. The standard time allotted to a visit is six to ten minutes per person, for regular complaints. Sometimes doctors will see patients for longer, depending on the seriousness of the case, but this longer visit must be booked in advance.

Janine and her five-year-old daughter, Wendy, often had the sniffles, especially in the winter. Janine wondered if she could do something to reduce the number of colds. Before trying alternative medicines, she wanted first to consult with her doctor. When she made an appointment for Wendy's regular checkup, she mentioned to the receptionist that she had some concerns she wanted to discuss.

After the checkup, Janine began to talk about her interest in alternative medicines. Her doctor appeared to be listening, but after a couple of minutes she looked at her watch, closed the file on her desk, and stood up.

"Sorry, Janine," she said. "I have other patients who need to see me. Can we talk about this at another visit?"

Janine was annoyed that the doctor did not appear to want to listen to her. She felt rushed, especially since she thought she had booked extra time to see the doctor.

"Oh!" said Janine. "I mentioned when I made the appointment that I wanted to talk to you about preventing colds. I thought that meant I'd get more time with you."

"Really?" said the doctor. "Are you sure? My receptionist is usually pretty good about telling me these things. Let me check with her." She left the room for a moment. When she returned, she told Janine that her appointment had been set for a standard visit.

Surprised, Janine apologized for the misunderstanding. "I guess I didn't make it clear enough. I'll make another appointment with you so we can talk. I really want your advice on herbal methods for reducing the number of colds we get."

"That's a good idea, Janine," said the doctor. "There's a lot to talk about."

Janine chose to express her dissatisfaction about feeling rushed immediately in a polite and open manner. Only through communicating did she realize that the dissatisfaction came from her error in not requesting a longer time with the doctor. Her assertiveness probably prevented a build-up of resentment and any misunderstandings with the doctor.

5.4 Feeling violated

When the situation goes beyond dissatisfaction, such as with a doctor's inappropriate behavior (or professional misconduct), there are serious steps that you can consider. If a doctor behaves inappropriately (e.g., sexual gestures, intimidation, or rude behavior), you need to first leave this doctor, then discuss the complaint with another professional at the complaints committee of the hospital or the Royal College of Physicians and Surgeons assigned to your area.

Susie's story is an extreme example. She had been seeing her doctor for about five years when the doctor's behavior seemed to change toward her. She spent more time than usual with Susie, and her conversation became friendlier. Susie didn't mind, in part, because she found the doctor interesting as a person. She also didn't suspect anything unusual in her friendliness.

Susie booked an appointment to discuss her recent breakup with her boyfriend. She was feeling emotionally vulnerable and needed to talk through some issues. The visit started out as usual: The doctor sat across from Susie and listened to her. When Susie started to feel a little emotional, the doctor reached out and held her hand. Susie was surprised, but she appreciated the gesture. As she talked more she found herself getting more emotional, and the doctor handed her a tissue to wipe her tears. She moved her chair close to Susie's and put her arm around her. Susie was uncomfortable, but she was too upset at the time to respond. When the visit was over, the doctor suggested Susie come back the next week, and Susie assumed the doctor's behavior was just an expression of support.

At the next visit, Susie became emotional again. This time when she began to cry, the doctor hugged her close. Susie felt herself stiffen. Then the doctor pressed her cheek against Susie's neck. Susie, startled, pulled away.

"Doctor!" she said. "I don't like what you're doing!"

"I don't know what you are talking about," said the doctor, coolly.

"You're getting too close to me!" said Susie.

The doctor became angry and told Susie that she was imagining things. This only made Susie certain that there was something wrong with the doctor's behavior. "Doctor, I know what happened," she said, her tears now gone. "This is the second time your behavior has been inappropriate."

"You couldn't be more wrong," said the doctor.

Susie left the office feeling very confused and hurt. She liked her doctor; she had respected and trusted her doctor. She didn't talk to anyone about how she felt right away. Finally she confided in a friend, who suggested she make a formal complaint.

With mixed feelings, Susie filed a complaint with the Royal College of Physicians and Surgeons. It took a long time for the complaint process to be completed, which was hard on Susie, but in the end she knew she had done the right thing (it turned out there had been one other similar complaint).

Approaching a doctor with concerns of dissatisfaction can be intimidating at any time, no matter how old or self-assured you are. Every situation has its degrees of dissatisfaction, and each can be handled differently, with different outcomes. An ethical doctor will always respond to your concerns attentively and professionally, even though it might be uncomfortable. This is when your good communication skills are especially useful. If you do not feel confident enough to confront the doctor, ask someone you trust to come with you. Consider your approach very carefully. Then, take action.

5.5 Feeling satisfied

Just as it's important to let the doctor know when you're dissatisfied, it's good to express your satisfaction, too. Part of feeling satisfied with a doctor is being aware that the doctor is supportive and sensitive to your needs. When those needs are met, let the doctor know.

All year Petra had aches and pains in her left shoulder and arm that prevented her from functioning well on a daily basis. She frequently went to see her doctor, sometimes in tears. He always supported her and searched to find a solution to her persistent pain. He talked to her, sent her for tests and x-rays, researched medical papers, and, finally, decided that she had bursitis.

"Petra," the doctor said, "I think we can solve this now." He explained everything he could about the condition and how to treat it. Then he said, "There is a medication that can help reduce the pain."

"At least I have a name for what I have," responded Petra. "I appreciate your time and support so much, doctor. I really feel you've done your best and I can't thank you enough for that."

"Thank you," replied the doctor. "Just your appreciation is enough. Having a patient who at least expresses some positive feedback is worth a lot to me."

Support at any level from your doctor offers you and the doctor both a sense of satisfaction. Whether the support is for you or for someone else, it is gratifying to know that you can call on this person to help you when you are in need. There are doctors who extend themselves beyond their daily service, in part, because it offers them personal reward. They don't have to extend themselves this way, but if you do have a doctor who has a warmth and inclination toward service beyond the call of duty, then you are fortunate. It is at this time that your expression of appreciation is welcomed.

As an example, one morning Dixie decided to take her two year-old son, Joshua, to the doctor. He had been listless and congested since the day before, and he had an upset stomach. Dixie left a message on the doctor's answering service asking if he had a space in his schedule to see Joshua. Later that morning, the doctor's receptionist called with an appointment.

When Dixie arrived, she had Joshua and his one-year-old sister, Olivia, with her. The doctor gave Joshua a thorough examination. The diagnosis was flu. Then the doctor suggested he take a look at Olivia too, so he checked her for similar symptoms, but she was all right. While he was explaining to Dixie what to do for Joshua, the little boy threw up. Dixie was embarrassed, but the doctor remained calm and was very patient with him.

The next day the doctor called Dixie to see how Joshua was feeling. His professional concern made her feel completely confident in him. She sent him a thank-you note to say how much she appreciated the extra care he took with her and her family.

Effective communication with your doctor benefits you in many ways. You create an open atmosphere for exchanging information, and offer insights into the state of your well-being, so you help your doctor to meet your needs. This is equally important when you're acting on behalf of others who can't communicate for themselves, for one reason or another, which we will discuss in the next chapter. In a way, good communication is part of taking care of yourself and your family.

Use Checklist 11 to rate the quality of your communication with your doctor, and to identify where it needs improving.

Checklist 11
Do You Communicate with Your Doctor Effectively?

Check yes or no for the answer that best describes you.

Question	Yes	No
Do you offer your doctor a complete medical history of yourself?		
Can you find words to describe your symptoms and how you feel?		
Do you get your point across?		
Do you make lists of questions to ask your doctor?		
Do you understand the advice your doctor gives you?		
Do you negotiate with your doctor when you have differing opinions?		
Do you tell your doctor if you are dissatisfied with the care you receive?		
Do you feel satisfied with the service your doctor provides?		

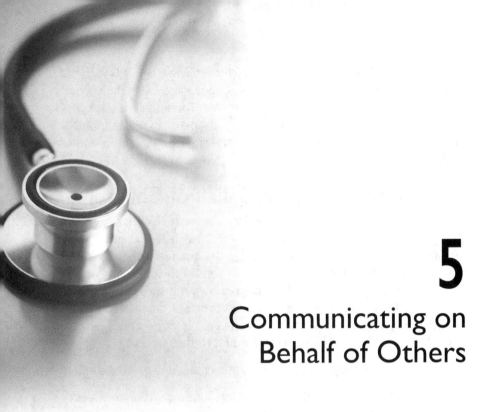

5

Communicating on Behalf of Others

Communicating on behalf of others is not always easy. It involves being acutely aware of someone else's needs and wants. Sometimes it's a guessing game; other times you might be especially aware of the other person's needs and wants.

You might be communicating for others who can't articulate their own thoughts, or they might not have enough language skills or reasoning to express their feelings accurately. Perhaps they're aware and conscious, but not willing or able to communicate. Perhaps there is a language barrier between the person and the doctor.

Your role, then, is to decipher and explain the other person's needs and wants to the doctor. You must depend on your understanding of the person's nonverbal communication such as crying, squirming, facial expressions, and any other physical expressions. More than likely, if you are speaking on behalf of someone close, you already have a sense of the meaning of that person's gestures; you might be expected to translate his or her symptoms or complaints to the doctor. Speaking on behalf of any other person requires a strong ability to listen to signals or suggestions.

When communicating on behalf of others, whether it is a friend, relative, or spouse, respect that person's needs and wants by consulting together before meeting with the doctor. Then be sure to express the needs and wants of that person to the doctor in a clear, concise manner, and relate the doctor's exact instructions or explanations back to the person.

1. Communicating on Behalf of Children

Anyone who spends time with children understands that there are times when a child's signals of discomfort are clear and other times when these signals are vague. Your ability to communicate for the child depends on understanding the signals as well as the closeness of your relationship with the child and the degree of seriousness of the child's complaint. To some extent this also draws on your familiarity with the child's ability to express verbally or non-verbally any fears of being ill and, of course, that ability varies according to the child's age.

Here are some suggestions for communicating on behalf of children:

- Make a list of the child's complaints and symptoms, with accurate and complete descriptions.

- Allow the child to do the talking if he or she is old enough.

- Listen closely to what the child says to the doctor.

- Support or add to the information the child says.

- Include older children in discussions with the doctor.

1.1 Younger children

You might only be able to describe things that may reflect symptoms such as a facial rash, runny nose, or crying. Identifying these specific signs will help the doctor assess the infant's discomfort.

However, once children are able to speak, they can respond directly to the doctor's questions. The adult's role, in this case, is to add support and any further description to the child's information. When Cathy took her three-year-old, Spencer, to the doctor, he asked the child questions and let Cathy fill in the gaps.

"How are you feeling today, Spencer?" asked the doctor.

"I don't feel good."

"Does it hurt somewhere?"

Spencer nodded.

"Can you show me where it hurts?" asked the doctor.

Spencer looked at his mother, who pointed to her throat.

"Is your throat sore?" asked the doctor.

"Yes," Spencer said. "Sore."

"Spencer woke up crying last night because his throat was sore," said Cathy. "He was a little feverish too, and he hasn't been able to eat any solid food in the last couple of days."

"Spencer," asked the doctor, "can you drink juice or eat yogurt?"

Spencer nodded.

"I have some special medicine to give you that will make your throat feel better," said the doctor, smiling. "Your mummy will give it to you in the morning and in the nighttime, okay?"

"Okay," said Spencer, looking at his mother for confirmation.

"I guess it'll take a few days before it helps, right?" asked Cathy.

"No, it should start to work within 24 hours."

As a parent or caregiver, it is helpful to both the child and the doctor if you can describe and confirm the child's responses to discomfort, as Cathy did.

1.2 Older children

An older child may be able to explain symptoms to the doctor and answer questions. In this situation, you can confirm those symptoms and negotiate a treatment plan for the child. What if you and your partner don't agree on a treatment plan? In the case of 12-year-old Michael, his parents had to negotiate with the doctor until they found a solution that satisfied all of them.

Michael had difficulty paying attention at school. His parents, Jack and Suzanne, consulted with the doctor about placing Michael on Ritalin or another drug prescribed for attention deficit hyperactivity disorder (ADHD).

Jack didn't see medication as a solution. He thought his son's inattention had to do more with being bored. He also did not want to see his son placed on drugs, as he put it.

Suzanne believed the drug treatment would be the solution to Michael's attention deficit and, since she usually helped Michael with his homework, she thought it would alleviate their frustration with his slow progress.

The doctor was sympathetic to the parents' concerns about Michael's poor performance at school. He started the discussion by asking Jack and Suzanne to describe their concerns.

Jack started. "I don't think Michael's problem is chemical," he said. "I think he's just bored … the classroom atmosphere doesn't fulfill his needs, so he gets bored and then acts out his frustration by cracking jokes or not paying attention. I know," he said, forcefully, "I've talked to him about this, and he is my son!"

"Suzanne, what are your thoughts on this?"

"He is my son, too," she said, looking directly at Jack. "I help Michael every night with his homework and I can see he has difficulty concentrating." She turned back to the doctor and continued. "Jack lets him watch far too much television when he gets home from school. I get home later, so I can't monitor his TV watching."

"That's not true!" said Jack. "We watch maybe half an hour, an hour max, before she gets home. We always have to wait for her."

"Jack, it is true," said Suzanne angrily, "and you know it!"

"What about Michael?" asked the doctor. "Have you asked him what he thinks about the idea of taking a drug?"

"Yes," said Jack quickly. "He doesn't want to take it."

"I wonder why?" Suzanne said, "you keep filling his head with reasons why he shouldn't. I read somewhere, doctor, that sometimes a blind study can help determine if a child has an attention deficit hyperactivity disorder. Do you know anything about this?"

"Yes, this is a possibility," said the doctor. "First we should have Michael come into the office so I can assess the situation with him."

"What's a blind study?" asked Jack.

"Michael would take different medications each day over a week or two," explained the doctor. "Each day he'd tell you how he feels, and you keep a record. No one knows which drug he is taking on any given day so there's no bias. At the end of the specified period, we'd look at the record to see the effect of the medication on Michael. What do you think about that, Jack?"

"I'm not sure," he said, looking at Suzanne. "It doesn't sound as bad as just placing him on one drug without any real evidence. I guess if Michael agrees, we can try it."

Michael, at the age of 12, had to be consulted, in part to engage his cooperation. Michael agreed to a blind study, and after two weeks they were able to determine that Ritalin did not improve his attention problem. Jack and Suzanne discussed non-medicated approaches with the doctor and, because of the willingness of everyone involved to consider all the options, they found a solution. Although his parents began in opposing camps, they were able to put Michael's well-being first. Their desire to explore options for their son allowed them to communicate effectively on his behalf.

2. Communicating on Behalf of the Elderly

Many of us have aging parents or relatives who are not necessarily ill but are slowing down. They might be very aware of their surroundings and those around them, but they might be unable to hear, see, or walk very well. As a result, they depend on us for any number of things, such as acting as their ears or eyes, relying on our ability to articulate for them, and counting on our memory. Of course they depend on our physical help and emotional support. Sometimes, however, we might not understand some of their behavior and might be unsure what to do.

Here are some suggestions for communicating on behalf of elderly people:

- Inform the doctor or medical office assistant of the nature of your visit.

- Inform the elderly person of the nature of the visit to the doctor.

- Make a list of the symptoms or concerns, with clear descriptions.

- Let the person speak, if possible.

- Listen carefully to everything the doctor says.

- Clarify the doctor's information by paraphrasing.

- Be sensitive to the elderly person's needs and wants.

- Ask the doctor to write down any instructions.

2.1 When couples communicate for one another

Albert and Agnes have been married for 50 years. When they visit the doctor, each remembers for the other. Each claims to know exactly what the other will say or how the other is feeling at all times. Their daughter Janet, worried about her parents' unusual way of communicating, called their doctor.

"If you listen to them, they sound as if they live in each other's head," explained Janet. "It's difficult to get a straight answer from either of them about their own health. It worries me, so I'd like you to assess them."

"Sounds interesting," said the doctor. "Why don't the three of you come in next week?"

When the appointment arrived, Janet accompanied her parents to the doctor's office. The doctor began by asking Albert and Agnes how they were doing.

"I'm very well, thank you," said Albert, "but Agnes is not feeling that good."

"What seems to be the problem, Agnes?"

"I'm not quite sure," said Agnes. "Bert says I've been tossing in my sleep."

"Yes, she has that sore knee again," said Albert. "You know, the one she had last summer ... it feels bruised and she seems to have difficulty walking on it, especially toward evening."

"Is that the way it feels, Agnes?" asked the doctor.

"I guess ... doesn't it Bert?"

"Yep, that's what it seems like."

Janet looked at the doctor. He nodded and turned to Agnes.

"Tell me, Agnes, how's Albert doing?"

"Oh, he's doing well," said Agnes, "except his coughing sometimes is a worry."

"What kind of a cough is it, Bert?" asked the doctor.

"Ask her!" said Albert. "She's the one who listens to it."

"It is sputtering, not very loud, just irritating. It wakes me up sometimes."

"Does the cough wake you up, too, Albert?" asked the doctor.

"Not usually, no."

"Yes, it does," said Agnes, "but not all the time." Janet shook her head.

"Well, if she says so," said Albert. "So I cough a little at night. I don't really remember."

After the visit, the doctor explained to Janet that although sometimes the interaction between Agnes and Albert seemed confusing, there was no harm in them communicating on behalf of one another.

"They're just taking care of each other," he said. "They spend a lot of time together. Who better to explain and remember how the other is doing. You know, your father said it well. He said, 'Agnes remembers for me because she looks after me, and I remember for her because I look after her.'"

"It sounds like they are fine with each other?" Janet asked.

"Absolutely," said the doctor. "In fact, this isn't unusual with people who've lived together for so long. They grow to depend on each other over the years, and they develop their own way of doing things. They develop their own understanding of what each other means."

As long as her parents' explanation remained clear and realistic, continued the doctor, Janet's responsibility was to offer support. If they reached a point when they could no longer depend on each other, she would then take on the role of communicating on their behalf. Meanwhile, Agnes and Albert appeared to be doing a good job of observing for each other.

2.2 When the issue is more than just health

Sometimes, as a guardian or personal caregiver, you may have to take the lead in finding alternative solutions to create a better quality of life, especially if you have the time and research skills to find alternatives.

Meredith's elderly parents live in a nursing home. Both Meredith's parents had failing sight as well as limited mobility. Her father also had loss of hearing and mild depression. He complained about not being in control, and as he so firmly stated, "I want to die." Meredith's mother, in contrast, had a higher energy level and more time on her hands plus a desire to socialize with the other ladies in the nursing home. Meanwhile, as her husband's depression increased, so did his memory lapses.

Meredith took a lead in searching for solutions. First she researched recent information on vitamin therapy for depression and concentration problems. After her search, she suggested to her father's doctor that perhaps injections of vitamin B12 would help improve her father's condition. The doctor agreed, prescribing injections every three weeks. Meredith said, "Thank goodness the doctor listened. My father's mental clarity improved soon after. He is a much happier person, and so is everyone around him."

When you are in a position to contribute to solutions for an aging person's quality-of-life issues, your best approach is to explore resources and updated medical information first before consulting with the doctor about your views on what you think needs to be done to help the patient. With evidence in hand, you will capture the doctor's attention more readily than if you argumentatively present informal ideas about the best medical cure-all.

2.3 Communicating on behalf of someone with hearing loss

Some people must hear and translate information for an adult whose hearing has gotten worse with age. At times this can be frustrating, especially if the person is in denial that there is any hearing loss. Even getting that person to be seen by a doctor might meet with a backlash of further denial. "Mind your own business," the person might say. "I don't have a problem!" In such instances, you might have to persuade the person in a roundabout way that it's time for a routine checkup.

Once there, the doctor might have better luck in persuading the elderly person to consider a hearing aid, if this is the solution to the problem. Your supportive presence is useful, especially since you can bring up the subject of the hearing loss and the patient's denial, such as Fred did when he accompanied his mother to the doctor's office.

"Doctor," said Fred. "I felt it was a good idea for my mother to have a routine checkup."

The doctor turned to Diana and asked, "What do you think of that, Diana?"

"Sorry, doctor, I wasn't paying attention," said Diana. "Could you repeat that?"

"Sure," said the doctor. In a clear, loud voice, he asked, "How are you today?"

"Fine, just fine," answered Diana. "No complaints. But my son here seems to think I am losing my hearing. I hear you perfectly well!"

"I'm just concerned about you, mother," said Fred.

"Doctor, I've noticed that I often have to repeat myself, and she turns the TV up louder than she used to."

"I see," said the doctor. "Are there any other concerns you have about your mother?"

"She doesn't always eat that well."

"All right, Diana, let's check your hearing and a few other things, and take a look at how you're doing," said the doctor. "Can you please step over here onto the scale so we can check your weight? Fred, perhaps you could take a seat in the waiting room while I complete the exam."

"You don't need me?" asked Fred. "I can interpret anything she doesn't understand."

"I think we'll manage," said the doctor, smiling at Diana. "I know where to find you if I need you."

Fred's idea of getting his mother to the doctor and asking the doctor to assess her hearing had its benefits. He was able to make sure the doctor would not rely only on the information Diana provided. The doctor could interact directly with her and address the issue of her hearing loss. At the end of the exam, he invited Fred back into the office, and together they discussed some of the hearing-aids available to her. The doctor also referred Diana to an audiologist to determine the extent of her hearing loss.

2.4 When an elderly person has concerns

Sometimes, the person for whom you are speaking might express discomfort with his or her relationship with the doctor. On such occasions, it is best to listen to the details of why the person feels this way. Regardless of the reason, you might want to address the concern with the doctor to form your own opinion.

You might already have some idea of the doctor's interaction style and approach to health care. Your impressions can provide a balanced view of the situation. Remember, however, that the patient is usually alone with the doctor so that person's impressions count first.

When someone complains or refuses to see the doctor, it might be a matter of a personality conflict, a misperception of the doctor's approach, denial about a health problem, or, especially in the case of elderly people, an indication of dementia. Whatever the reason, you and the person need to discuss an alternative choice of a doctor.

Dan's father complained repeatedly about his doctor. Dan wondered if his father just did not like his doctor's personality. He asked his father for his impressions of the doctor.

"The way he handles me during the exam hurts. He's too strong," said Norm. "It's not just when he touches me; it's also the way he talks to me. He's rude. I don't even think he bothers to listen to me."

Dan was concerned. He wanted Norm to see the doctor for his bronchitis, which had flared up again. Dan offered to accompany him to the doctor, and his father agreed. This would give Dan a chance to observe the doctor's interaction style and compare it to his father's views. When they arrived at the doctor's office, the doctor asked Norm to describe how he was feeling, and Dan listened to the two men talk. After a while, Dan turned to Norm and said, "Dad, I'd like to tell the doctor what you told me about coming to see him. Do you mind, or would you like to tell him?"

"You tell him," said Norm, looking a little uncomfortable.

"Would you like to stay here," asked Dan, "or sit in the waiting room?"

"I'll wait outside."

After his father left the room, Dan began by telling the doctor that Norm had told him he was sometimes left alone in the examining room for 45 minutes before anyone came to see him. "Is this normal?" asked Dan. "Are people usually left alone that long?"

"I wouldn't say it's normal," answered the doctor. "Sometimes there's a backlog of patients so the wait can get quite lengthy."

"I see," said Dan. "My father also told me he is uncomfortable with your manner."

"Oh?" said the doctor. "What does he mean?"

"He tells me that you do not consult him about treating his cough," said Dan. "He also feels that when you examine him that you are too rough. Is that possible?"

"Do you know what he means by that?" asked the doctor.

"Yes, I do." Dan listed the examples of the doctor's behavior that Norm had told him. Norm had described two specific incidents to him, so Dan was able to give the doctor detailed information.

"Thank you for telling me this, Dan," said the doctor, thoughtfully. "I'll make a point of involving him more, such as asking him how he feels about the treatment plan. As for being rough, this is the first time I've received such a complaint. I will take special care to be more gentle with Norm. How about we get him back in here so we can complete the exam?"

He went to the door and called Norm to come back into the office. Dan excused himself and went to wait for his father in the waiting room. On the way home, Dan asked Norm how the rest of the visit went. Norm said the doctor asked him more questions, which he appreciated. This time, instead of taking his arm and guiding him on to the examining table like he usually did, the doctor asked Norm if he needed help. When this had happened before, Norm had thought the doctor was pushing him around because he had no confidence in the older man. However, the doctor's question made him realize that the doctor was trying to be helpful.

Dan listened to his father. He observed that these issues could be discussed comfortably with the doctor, and they could produce a positive result. Norm agreed, and decided to remain with his doctor.

3. Communicating on Behalf of Someone Who Is Terminally Ill

Communicating on behalf of someone who is terminally ill can be exhausting. Perhaps you have been assigned medical and financial power of attorney so you are legally entrusted with overseeing the personal health and financial affairs of a loved one. This responsibility requires you to juggle life's ever-demanding activities including communicating the person's wants and needs to the doctor.

You also need to remember to look after yourself, which includes taking time to talk with people who can offer you personal and moral support.

3.1 When the person is in denial about dying

When someone is in denial of impending death, consider asking the doctor for guidance on the best way to handle the situation. You might also need to communicate any changes or improvements you see in the patient's outlook or condition.

When Gary's wife, Linda, was ill with breast cancer, he became the sole source of support for her and their children. In the beginning stages of the disease Linda fell into denial, and then anger. She claimed that there must be some mistake in the test results.

At first Linda demanded that Gary ask another doctor to double-check the results of her tests. Gary would make all the necessary arrangements, and accompany her to all the appointments. It was a difficult time for him because he wasn't sure what was happening to their lives, but Linda was too defiant to discuss their future in any reasonable way. He felt as if they were in some kind of surreal state. Even he pretended that the disease would go away. Finally, he made an appointment to discuss the situation with Linda's doctor at the hospital. He told the doctor that he and Linda were having a rough time dealing with her illness.

"Is this really happening to us?" asked Gary. "Is Linda really going to die?"

"Linda has advanced breast cancer," explained the doctor, "which can be treated with chemotherapy. That will probably prolong her life by about six months."

"Six months ... That can't be true," said Gary. "I was so sure the treatments were working."

"We're all doing the best we can," said the doctor. "However, we can't deny the sad facts, I'm afraid. We want to help you both get through this rough time, and help you make peace with this situation."

"Peace?" cried Gary. "Peace? Why should I feel peaceful about losing my wife? Why is this happening to her?"

"Anger is a natural reaction, Gary," said the doctor, "as is denial, for both of you. But it's important for you to understand the facts and to help her as best you can."

"I try, doctor. I'd do anything for Linda," said Gary. "However, nothing I do seems to work. She seems so angry and sad all the time, and often she won't even admit that there's anything seriously wrong with her. What can I do?"

"I know," said the doctor sympathetically. "It sounds like you're doing a terrific job already. She needs to know she can count on your support. Tell her you love her and stay by her side as much as you can." He reached into his desk for some handouts. "You know, there are several support groups here in town that can help you through this process. They can help you find the words and strength to support her. There are even some support groups on this list that Linda might consider attending, too."

"That's a good idea, doctor. Maybe if she sees other women like her ... "

"Yes, support groups can go a long way to helping people cope."

Gary started to feel very emotional. "Yesterday she suddenly turned to me and said, 'Will it be painful in the end?'" He started to cry softly. "What do I tell her?"

"Gary, just reassure her as best you can. I will talk to her directly about these things. I'd also like to talk to you both together. Can you both meet me here tomorrow afternoon?"

"I'll try," replied Gary, blowing his nose. "I can't promise. Sometimes Linda gets really angry that no one can stop the disease from getting worse. Can I let you know in the morning?"

"Yes, of course," said the doctor. "I'll expect your call."

Gary registered that afternoon with one of the support groups at the hospital, which helped him learn how to deal with his own feelings about the changes in his life as well as Linda's. As Linda's health deteriorated, she relied more heavily on Gary to communicate her needs and wants to the doctor. With the help of their health-care team and the fellow members of his support group, Gary was able to guide his wife toward a death with dignity. Even after Linda passed away, Gary continued to talk with the doctor for a few weeks as well as attend the support group.

3.2 When the person wants to die at home

As a caregiver, maintaining your own stamina depends on your health, your ability to make decisions, and your skill in communicating with a variety of people about matters that are sometimes very emotionally charged. Keeping an open perspective about the needs of the person you're caring for is paramount, especially when that person wants to go home to die.

It's natural to want to provide comfort for someone who is terminally ill. Your knowledge of that person's desires is invaluable when you have to decide how to do that. This might require a prior written document or verbal statement by the person confirming any preferences for treatment in the end stages of illness. Or perhaps the person is able to participate in the choice of where to die. In any case, your role in the decision should be based on your personal knowledge of the individual and his or her condition.

However, the final decision might be met with resistance from the doctor or a palliative care team. In such situations, good communication skills, such as listening, expressing yourself assertively, and negotiating, will be useful.

Caroline had to decide whether her aunt Arlet would be most comfortable in the final stages of stomach cancer in the hospital or at home. The older woman was expected to live for another five or six weeks. She knew from conversations with Arlet before she became seriously ill that she preferred to remain at home in the end stages of the disease. The specialist recommended that Arlet stay at a palliative care facility, where she felt Arlet's needs would be better met.

Although the decision was ultimately Caroline's and her aunt's, Caroline was confused about what to do. Caroline felt strongly about respecting her aunt's wishes. She decided to consult with her aunt's

GP, whom Arlet had been seeing for 20 years. She explained her dilemma to the doctor, who agreed that Arlet would be more comfortable at home.

"I feel so pressured by the specialist to have her placed in a palliative care facility," said Caroline. "She's got a point; she says the facility is better equipped to deal with Arlet's needs, and that it will be less draining on me. I really think Aunt Arlet wants to come home. Could you call the specialist for me?"

"It's not usual for the GP to intervene at this stage," said the doctor.

"I want to respect her wishes!" said Caroline. "I've listened to the specialist's reasons, and I've discussed this with you. I really think the thing to do is to let Arlet come home. We can bring in some professional help if we need to."

"All right," said the GP. "I happen to know that specialist well so I'll see what I can do. I'll let you know the outcome in a couple of days."

Caroline's aunt passed away comfortably in her own home, and Caroline never regretted her decision.

4. Communicating on Behalf of People with Language and Cultural Barriers

Imagine traveling alone in a foreign land surrounded by people who don't speak your language. How does it feel when you need directions or want to buy food and no one understands you? How does it feel when someone asks you a question but you can't make sense of what is being asked?

Now imagine these feelings in the context of needing health care. You might feel lost or frightened because everyone around you is different from what you know. There might be some similarities in customs, values, and attitudes, but the language might be different from your own. You want someone to understand your immediate needs, but you don't know how to communicate them.

Imagine what it must be like in this situation when you need someone to help you with your pain.

Here are some suggestions for communicating on behalf of someone who has a language barrier:

- Let the doctor know before the appointment that the person speaks a different language.

- Explain what to expect at the doctor's office to the person.

- Ask the person to explain any symptoms or concerns to you before the doctor visit, and make a detailed list.

- Translate the person's description of discomfort accurately.

- Explain in detail the doctor's comments or instructions to the person.

- Ask the person if there are any further questions for the doctor.

4.1 When language and culture barriers exist

People who have recently arrived in North America might speak very little English, Spanish, or French. Often in these cases, a relative or community volunteer who speaks the newcomer's language might act as an interpreter. Sometimes the person understands enough of what is said to interact independently with the doctor, but the customs and procedures might be very unfamiliar.

Suha took her 60-year-old mother to her GP because of severe pain resulting from rheumatoid arthritis. Najat was shy and uncomfortable about seeing a doctor in a foreign country. It had not occurred to Suha at the time to meet with the doctor a few minutes beforehand. Najat understood some of the information exchanged between her daughter and the doctor, who recommended a number of gold injections as a treatment. After several months, Najat still found the pain unbearable so Suha returned with her to consult with the doctor.

"Doctor, what can my mother expect from long-term treatment?" Suha asked.

"The pain she is experiencing is something she will have to learn to live with," he said.

The doctor's blunt delivery of information upset Suha. Having lived in North America for 15 years, she was accustomed to the different style of communication from her country of origin, but she knew her mother would be intimidated by such straightforwardness. Najat was also upset, because she understood enough to grasp the meaning of what the doctor had said, but she did not know how to respond.

As they left the doctor's office, Suha realized she should have met with the doctor alone for a few minutes before the visit. This would have been a good opportunity for Suha to let the doctor know of the cultural conventions Najat was used to, and they could have discussed ways of informing her mother appropriately of the long-term prognosis.

4.2 Overcoming the language and culture gap

Steve, a US citizen, developed pains in his right side while traveling in rural Quebec, Canada, with his girlfriend, Alyssa (Canadian descent, with a French-speaking mother). She wanted Steve to see a doctor, but neither of them spoke French. She convinced Steve to go to a community health center near where they were staying. While they were waiting, his pain worsened, and it was up to Alyssa to try to provide most of the background information to the receptionist. All Steve could do was groan, although his facial expression needed no translation.

When they got into the doctor's office, Alyssa said the only French phrase she remembered from childhood: "Je ne parle pas français." ("I don't speak French.") The doctor tried to communicate with hand gestures and the few words in English he knew. Alyssa did the same, gesturing toward Steve. The doctor understood that Steve's pain was mainly in his lower abdominal area.

Alyssa noticed a picture of the human body in the doctor's office. She pointed to the location of the exact area. Somehow, she managed to understand that the doctor needed to know how long Steve had been in pain. She put her hands together and laid her cheek on them, with her eyes closed, to indicate that Steve had been sleeping. Then she held up two fingers and then pointed to the clock with a counter-clockwise motion to try to indicate the pain had started two hours before he went to bed the previous night. The doctor was able to piece together what Alyssa told him with the results of his examination of Steve to diagnose his condition.

When there is a language barrier, nonverbal communication might be the only means to get the message across. Alyssa used common sense when gesturing Steve's symptoms to the doctor. Steve's facial expression also showed the depth of his pain. Both helped to convey valuable information to the doctor. Even without words, Alyssa and Steve provided essential information to the doctor.

However, common gestures in one culture might be interpreted differently in another. For example, silence can be interpreted as agreement in one culture and disagreement in another. A particular tone of voice might reflect annoyance in one culture, but something else in another. Speaking loudly might send a message of anger, when the intention is excitement. In many cultures, not looking someone in the eye is a sign of respect; in others, it means disrespect.

Certain personal behavior can also have different meanings. A direct stare or minimal eye contact might represent personal style and not mood. Someone's cool glance or warm smile might display something other than what we initially interpret. Any one of these patterns of communication might influence how you and the doctor interpret one other.

Keep in mind that there are universal or general gestures that are understood by everyone, no matter what the cultural background. Do not hesitate, however, to use your own personal nonverbal gestures to explain how you feel to the doctor. The aim here as always is to try to be clear and simple in your communication to enable the doctor to give the best of care.

Here are some suggestions for communicating nonverbally:

- Use simple gestures and simple facial, hand, and body movements.

- Make sounds to express discomfort.

- Remember that a gesture might mean one thing to you and another thing to someone else.

- Use pictures or point to the specific area on the body to show pain or discomfort.

- Observe the patient's gestures to decipher any discomfort.

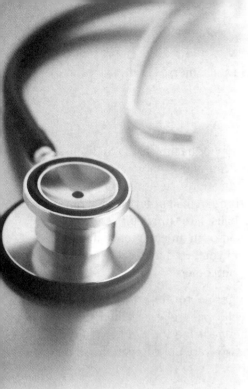

6
Beyond the Routine Checkup

We've seen the importance of good communication in standard patient-doctor situations. Open communication becomes even more important when problems extend beyond the routine checkup, or in a health-care crisis. In these circumstances, you might have to consider different questions and communication strategies.

For instance, you will likely have questions about the drugs you are prescribed, the tests you are sent for, the specialist you see, the short- and long-term prognosis for the condition you have, or other questions appropriate to your situation. You might not be prepared with relevant questions on the spot, but you can ask the doctor general questions about the short- and long-term side effects of medications and about the necessity of rest or referral to a specialist.

Likewise, you might have many questions about causes of chronic health problems, such as fibromyalgia and chronic fatigue syndrome. However, in the case of some conditions, you're unlikely to get any concrete answers since research has yet to find their causes. Doctors are often more familiar with treating chronic illnesses that have established treatment plans.

1. Prescribed Drugs

One of the many ways of taking charge of your health care is to discuss with the doctor what medications you can and cannot take. Inform the doctor of any over-the-counter medications, health supplements (whether bought at a store or received through mail order), herbal remedies (even those recommended by herbalists), or drugs prescribed by another doctor such as a specialist, a doctor in an emergency department, or a naturopath. Doing so can help you avoid medical complications that could lead to serious or fatal outcomes.

For instance, when Rebecca visited her doctor for arthritic pain in her hip, the doctor recommended a specific pain reliever. When Rebecca asked how it would interact with the medicine she used to control her asthma, the doctor replied that the two were not compatible, so he chose another pain reliever.

The doctor had forgotten Rebecca had asthma, but Rebecca's record-keeping and awareness of drug interactions allowed her to avoid problematic side effects. This is why keeping a record of any medications you take gives both you and the doctor an opportunity to cross-check any prescriptions. It's always best to ask the doctor if the prescribed medication interacts with any other medications you are taking before getting the prescription filled.

Similarly, at the drugstore, always ask the pharmacist about potential side effects, check the labels and instructions for the amount of drug to take and at what time to take it. Ask if the prescribed drug comes in a generic brand, which is usually less expensive.

1.1 Drug reactions or side effects

By reminding the doctor of allergies or other side effects to certain medications, you can also help avoid a crisis. It's a good idea to bring your medication with you to appointments as a reminder. These practices help keep everyone on top of the types of medication prescribed for you and their side effects. Combining the information from your doctor and local pharmacist is a good start.

Doctors and pharmacists often consult one another about new drug remedies and drug interactions; pharmacists have at least four years of schooling focusing on the substance and quality of prescribed and over-the-counter medications. The general practitioner's education in this area is substantially less; in fact, they will mostly rely on the drug company's representative for the basic side effects and information on a particular medication. It is then up to the GP to learn more about it through sound medical research articles, for instance.

Discussing any drug intake with your doctor as well as your pharmacist reduces the risk of adverse side effects. Remember to mention whether you smoke tobacco and, if you drink alcohol or take illegal substances, ask what effect they might have on the effectiveness of the drug.

In Beverly's case, taking the initiative to tell her doctor immediately of specific adverse drug reactions probably saved her life. Not long after her cardiologist prescribed new medication for a chronic heart condition, her GP gave her a prescription for strong medication for migraines. When she took the first dose of the migraine medication, she began to feel heart palpitations. Concerned, she considered going to the local emergency department, but decided to contact her GP instead. The GP immediately identified the cause as a reaction to the migraine medication in combination with the new pills prescribed by the cardiologist for her heart condition. The cardiologist's report had not yet reached the GP's office so she had not known about the new medication. Also, it so happened that Beverly had not gone to her usual drugstore to have the prescription for the migraine medication filled; her regular pharmacist, who was familiar with her prescription history, would have noticed that it was incompatible with her heart medication.

Communicate the following information:

- Tell the pharmacist and doctor about all other prescription or over-the-counter medications you are taking, no matter who recommended or prescribed it.

- Tell the doctor if you are pregnant.

- Tell the doctor if you have allergies.

- Tell the pharmacist and doctor about any supplements or herbal remedies you are taking.

- Tell the doctor immediately of any adverse side effects or drug reactions.

- Tell yourself that having a regular pharmacist for consistent record-keeping is beneficial.

1.2 Over-the-counter drugs

Drugs sold over the counter (OTC) or behind the counter (BTC) require the same respect and consideration as any other drug. They can pose a serious threat when combined with other drugs.

All drugs are pharmaceutical substances, even those sold to treat common colds, pain, and allergies. They are developed and marketed by the same drug companies that make prescription drugs. These drugs contain amounts of active ingredients considered safe for self-treatment by consumers when the instructions are followed. Often drugs that once required a doctor's prescription become available over the counter or from behind the counter — sold by the pharmacist without a prescription.

We may not be aware of how OTC drugs may interact with a prescription drug. It is important, therefore, to discuss any OTC and prescription medicines you are planning to take with your pharmacist. Likewise, if you are planning an evening of entertainment involving a glass or two of wine or some other alcoholic beverage, ask the doctor or the pharmacist if the OTC medicine and alcohol can cause any adverse reactions.

Alexia's job required her to attend several luncheons a month. One day, on her way to a formal luncheon, she dropped by the pharmacy for something to get rid of piercing menstrual cramps. She purchased some extra strength anti-inflammatory pills and took a double dose. Alexia didn't bother to consult the pharmacist or read the label on the bottle, and she had never discussed pain relief with her doctor.

Seated at a table of high-profile businesspeople, Alexia had a glass of wine with her lunch. While talking to the CEO next to her, she began to feel woozy. She excused herself and went to the powder room, where she sat down with her head between her knees. After a few minutes, she stood up, picked up her purse from the counter, and started back toward the dining room. Suddenly, she fell back against the wall and slid to the floor, spilling the contents of her purse. Her vision was blurry and her head was swirling. Several people came over to help her and, when her head cleared a little, she took a taxi straight to her doctor's office (it may have been a better choice to go straight to the emergency room). The doctor asked her questions about what she had eaten, and when she mentioned the drugs and the wine, the doctor knew immediately what the problem was. Because Alexia was still feeling nauseous and dizzy, the doctor wasn't too hard on her, but he did make it clear to Alexia that her actions had been irresponsible. She should have checked whether the anti-inflammatory medicine would interact with alcohol.

Many other OTC drugs can cause similar adverse reactions, in some cases fatal. It only takes a couple of minutes to ask the pharmacist or read the label. It is also important to let your doctor know of OTC drugs you may take for headaches, menstrual cramps, backaches, or other common complaints. See Checklist 12. (You can print the following checklist by using the download kit instructions at the end of this book. Take the checklist with you to your doctor appointment or to the pharmacist and write down your answers for future reference.)

1.3 Staying with the regimen

People can fail to take their prescribed drugs for any number of reasons. These can include forgetfulness, confusion, resistance to being told what to do, or a dislike of being dependent on medications. If you have difficulty staying with a regimen for whatever reason, it is important to let your doctor know.

If a drug routine is a problem, the doctor might ask to see you on a weekly basis, especially if the prescription is a short-term daily dose. If the prescription is for a longer period, the doctor might suggest using a labeled plastic pill container that can be bought at any pharmacy.

When Jean, for instance, was first diagnosed as a diabetic, the doctor explained the importance of taking the pills to keep her sugar balanced. At first, she had a problem accepting the diagnosis of diabetes and didn't like the idea that she would have to take pills every day for the rest of her life. She told the doctor how she felt. As a result, he monitored her regularly until she got used to the routine and the idea of having diabetes.

Jean found that by explaining her concerns to the doctor she received the support she needed to adjust to the new routine, and she avoided any dire complications that might have occurred if she had not taken her medication. Keep in mind that not all doctors provide support services equally.

Communicate the following information:

- Tell the doctor if you feel uncomfortable taking a new drug.

- Tell the pharmacist of any new drugs that you need to take, whether for a short time or a long time.

- Ask the doctor or pharmacist if he or she will monitor your progress regularly at first.

- Ask the doctor or pharmacist to give you any updated information on drug interactions.

Checklist 12
Ask the Doctor or Pharmacist about Medications — Prescription and Over-the-Counter

Question	Answer
What is the difference between over-the-counter drugs, behind-the-counter drugs, and prescribed drugs?	
How can I avoid drug interactions?	
What drug am I taking?	
What is the drug designed to do?	
What are the short-term effects of this drug on my body?	
What side effects should I expect? What should I do about them?	
How and when should I take this drug?	
Should I take the drug with food or on an empty stomach?	
Should I avoid any foods, substances, or activities while taking the drug?	
How long should I take the drug?	
What should I do if I forget to take a dose?	
How long before my symptoms will improve?	
Does it come in a generic brand?	

2. When You Prefer Alternative Medicines or Therapies

Many people prefer alternative medical treatments for reducing discomfort or prolonging life today. These approaches often include mega doses of vitamins, herbal remedies, acupuncture, relaxation techniques, homeopathy, or other naturopathic remedies. Exercise or physical therapies, such as physiotherapy, massage, swimming, applying heat packs, and meditating, can be recommended under alternative ways to healing. For some people, these approaches are auxiliaries; that is, they support conventional treatments such as chemotherapy or prescription drugs. They might be an effective way to manage short-term or long-term side effects of conventional treatments. Sometimes people who prefer alternative approaches are discouraged by their medical doctor who might not have explored these treatment options. The patient or caregiver might also be poorly informed of the benefits of conventional treatments. In such cases, good communication between the doctor, caregiver, and patient is all the more important.

Rhoda's story is an interesting example. An uncertified but well-informed naturopath, she wanted her father to try some alternative medicines, such as a particular tree bark, to help prolong his life. He had pancreatic cancer, and had been told he had only a few weeks to live. She discussed the idea with her father and mother, and then mentioned it to the specialist.

"Perhaps you think that alternative medicines are superior to conventional medicines," the doctor said angrily. "You are wrong!"

"I don't think so," said Rhoda, remaining calm. "Besides, I've discussed this with my parents, and this is the approach my father would prefer."

The specialist remained convinced that Rhoda was wrong. Rhoda began to describe some of the research findings she had read on the approach she was suggesting. She explained that she had discussed this with her own GP, who was more open to alternative approaches. Eventually, he agreed to let her father try the remedy, but only after Rhoda produced an article she had been reading in a reputable magazine. It so happened that Rhoda's father actually lived a year and a half longer. Rhoda was sure that extra time was the result of the use of alternative medicines.

Rhoda's scenario is still a common occurrence. Because the Royal College of Physicians and Surgeons does not yet allow medical doctors to prescribe alternative medicines, few doctors educate themselves on alternative medicines or recommend them as part of a treatment plan. Medical schools also do not make course work in complementary medicine mandatory. (However, some medical school programs and teaching hospitals are beginning to be more open to including courses on alternative medicines as an option, especially in the United States.) Many doctors are too busy to read the masses of information produced from medical and health research. They must pick and choose what they can read. Therefore, it is difficult for a doctor to make an informed decision about the use of alternative medicines.

In many respects, it is up to you to research this information and educate yourself about respective conventional and alternative medicines. This takes time and effort, and a willingness to discuss options with conventional health-care professionals. (Some pharmacists have included in their service a software program or app that provides information to them on the side effects of alternative medicines with that of conventional prescribed medicines. Ask your pharmacist if he or she uses this program.)

Information comes from all sources. There are many legitimate Internet health websites with information about herbal remedies or homeopathy. There are also established health centers that offer advice on homeopathy and naturopathy. Perhaps you can ask a friend or relative to help you gather information. Consult with both your GP and a homeopathic or naturopathic practitioner about combination therapies primarily because some "health" websites are not qualified to provide medically viable information. This may be a reason that you receive opposition from both parties. Most prefer one approach over another, and will try to persuade you to do the same.

Rhoda handled the situation with her father's doctor effectively. She was able to negotiate with him because she had done her research. She had even brought materials along with her to support her argument. Had the specialist still resisted using alternative medicine, Rhoda could have sought a second opinion, but because she made a strong case on her own she didn't have to make that effort.

Keep in mind the following steps when promoting an alternative medicine approach to the doctor:

- Research evidence-based information about possible alternative health solutions.

- Summarize the facts and information about the treatment or approach when informing the doctor.

- Discuss your reasons for the alternative medicine approaches openly and clearly.

- Listen to the doctor's opinions, considering them as well as the alternative medicine approaches.

Communicate the following:

- Tell the doctor and pharmacist if you are considering taking homeopathic remedies, especially if you have been prescribed conventional drugs.

- Tell the doctor and pharmacist if you are pregnant.

- Tell the doctor and pharmacist if you have allergies.

- Tell the doctor and pharmacist if you have any side effects.

Don't forget to bring a list of your own questions and points to discuss with the doctor or pharmacist, depending on your own situation or condition. See Checklist 13.

Checklist 13
Questions to Ask a Homeopathic or Naturopathic Doctor or Pharmacist

Ask the following questions if you are seeing a homeopath or naturopath for the first time.

Question	Answer
What is difference between homeopathy and naturopathy?	
How have the remedies been tested?	
How do they work?	
What are the remedies made of?	
How does a particular alternative medicine compare to its counterpart in conventional medicine?	

3. When the Doctor Is Away

Doctors like their weekends or statutory holidays as much as you do. If you do not want to be left in the position of saying, "Oh, no, now what do I do?" when your prescription runs out unexpectedly, be proactive and ask your doctor to register a repeat prescription with the pharmacist. Without a prescription, the pharmacist is not authorized to give you any prescribed drug. Your doctor or the locum (replacement) must authorize it. If that's not possible, go to the closest emergency department. You must bring a labeled bottle of the last prescription filled to show the emergency doctor proof you are the person prescribed the medication.

Elaine's husband had severe arthritis and had recently been diagnosed with cancer. At this point, Elaine was taking care of him at home, including giving him prescribed injections of morphine for pain. Elaine suddenly realized late one Friday afternoon that she did not have enough morphine to last the next few days.

It was a long weekend, and the GP had already left the office. Elaine tried to persuade the pharmacist to release a repeat prescription, but he apologized, saying he could not authorize any medication without a doctor's permission. Elaine pleaded with the pharmacist. She only needed a small dose to tide her husband over, she said. Couldn't the pharmacist make an exception for someone in such pain? The pharmacist was familiar with Elaine and her husband's condition, and could hear the desperation in Elaine's voice. After some thought, he made a few phone calls and found the doctor who handled emergencies for Elaine's GP. He explained to Elaine that usually it is up to the patient to telephone the doctor who is on call, and that most GPs leave a recorded message with the contact information for emergencies. Under the circumstances, this time he made an exception and, with the permission of the on-call doctor, the pharmacist renewed the prescription.

Both Elaine and her husband were very grateful. Elaine realized that although the team made up of her, the pharmacist, and the on-call doctor moved things in a desirable direction, it was also her ability to explain the situation clearly to the pharmacist that brought about positive resolution. But she learned her lesson-from then on, she always made provisions for extra medication, and took special care with drugs such as the powerful painkillers her husband relied on.

Communicate the following:

- Tell the doctor that you need a repeat prescription.

- Tell the pharmacist about all the medications you are taking.

- Ask when the doctor or pharmacist will return.

- Ask for the telephone number of the on-call doctor.

4. When You Are Being Sent for Tests

There are common tests and not-so-common tests ordered by doctors. Both categories are selected for different reasons. We can guess that the common tests, which are widely used, are likely linked with our routine checkup and provide the doctor with general information about our health.

Not-so-common tests are generally ordered to investigate some kind of disease or abnormality. These tests often involve the use of expensive technology, such as magnetic resonance imaging (MRI), and technicians to operate them.

Then there are the unnecessary tests. Sometimes these are ordered for the sake of using expensive and new technology (the hospital administrators have to justify the use of the fancy equipment). Sometimes people, like Paulette, insist on having these tests done, despite evidence that no further investigation is needed.

Paulette visited her doctor frequently because of tension headaches. She usually managed the pain by taking over-the-counter drugs, but she was increasingly frustrated because the headaches wouldn't go away. Finally, on one visit, she told the doctor she could no longer stand the pain.

"What do you want me to do?" asked the doctor, who was also frustrated. "I've recommended just about everything for your problem. You have classic symptoms of a tension headache."

"There must be something really wrong," said Paulette. "I think I should have one of those brain scans to find out what it is."

"Do you mean a CAT scan? I really don't think that is necessary. There's one other possible treatment we could try. It involves an injection, though."

"No, no," said Paulette. "I want a CAT scan. If you won't order it, I'll just have to find a doctor who will, or I'll go to the emergency department or even a private clinic and pay out of pocket."

This put doctor in an awkward position. He was certain the CAT scan would reveal nothing. He didn't want to lose Paulette as a patient, and he didn't want her taking up time in an emergency department or wasting health-care costs for unnecessary tests. He tried to change her mind, but to no avail. Reluctantly the doctor ordered a scan and, as expected, the results came back as negative.

Although people may occasionally demand unnecessary tests, likewise a person may need to challenge the doctor to order specific tests to relieve suspicions of serious injury or disease. Similarly, the doctor may insist on unwarranted tests — here is an instance when you must seriously question whether such tests are a waste of time and cost to the health-care system.

Samantha slipped on wet cement steps, injuring her foot. Since she was a doctor, she knew she had broken a bone, but wasn't sure the extent of the damage. Even doctors need to see the doctor, and the one she consulted told her that the injury was a simple sprain. Samantha responded that she thought she had a hairline fracture and wanted an x-ray, but the GP insisted it was unnecessary.

"Look," said Samantha, "I am a doctor and I think I have a good sense of my own body too, and I insist that an x-ray is done!" She was frustrated that the doctor was not respecting her desires or recognizing what she thought was necessary.

"Fine, let's see what the results are," the doctor said with a shrug. Sure enough, the results showed a hairline fracture.

Raisa had persistent throbbing pain in her left side so she went to see her doctor. The doctor recommended an ultrasound to see what the problem was. Nervous, Raisa asked the doctor what it might be, but the doctor tried to reassure her by saying she couldn't be sure until the test results arrived. Raisa persisted until finally the doctor said that the problem could be an ovarian cyst.

Raisa's eyes widened. "Is this serious? How bad is it?"

"Raisa, we can't know anything until you have the test. It might not be a cyst. It might be nothing."

"If there's a cyst, you'd remove it right? Does that mean I'd have to have an operation?"

"If there really is a cyst, how we treat it depends on its size," said the doctor. "If it's about the size of a lemon, I'd probably recommend surgery, but if it's smaller, we might just let it dissolve by itself."

"You mean you'd do nothing?" Raisa asked.

"Cysts often form during ovulation. Let's do the test first before we jump to any hasty conclusions."

Raisa had the ultrasound, went home, and waited for two days for a call from the doctor's office. Even though her pain subsided, she was still worried. On the third day, she called the doctor's office. The medical office assistant said, "Oh, yes, Raisa, the results were in yesterday. Can you come in and see the doctor tomorrow?"

"Why didn't you call me if the test results were in yesterday?" asked Raisa. "I've been so worried!"

"I'm sorry. It's been really busy around here."

Raisa's fears were confirmed. The doctor recommended she see a surgeon to have an approximately two-inch (four-centimeter) cyst removed. "I thought that wouldn't be necessary unless the cyst was larger? Besides, I don't have any more pain."

The doctor persuaded Raisa to see the specialist. While she sat waiting for two hours, she had time to reconsider her decision and listen to her own instincts. She left the office. She returned to her GP and asked for another ultrasound to see if the cyst had dissolved. The doctor complied, and Raisa's theory was proven correct. The cyst had dissolved. In Raisa's case, she listened to her own body; she knew that the absence of pain meant something had changed.

In Melvin and Hilda's case, they listened to media reports on the latest research. They knew that recently developed technologies could help detect all kinds of risky conditions. Melvin's doctor had told him that the recurring pain in his left shoulder was caused by a chipped collarbone. Melvin and Hilda were concerned, and they thought more should be done, given what they had learned from watching health shows on television. So Hilda took Melvin to the doctor and insisted he have a MRI.

"I know you are concerned," said the doctor, "but an MRI is very costly to the health system. Melvin doesn't need to have an MRI to have his problem correctly diagnosed."

"Okay, doctor," Hilda said. "But if anything happens to my Melvin, you'll be hearing from me."

"All right, Hilda," replied the doctor. "I'm confident that there is no need for this test." A year later Melvin still had occasional pain, but it was well managed through medication with no further complications.

Communicate to the specialist the following:

- Tell the doctor if another doctor has recently tested you.

- Tell the doctor if you would like to explore alternative solutions to testing.

- Tell the doctor that you will call for the test results at an appropriate time.

- Tell the doctor if you feel the test is unnecessary.

You can print Checklist 14 by using the download link at the end of this book. Take the form with you to your appointment and write down the answers for later reference.

Checklist 14
What to Ask the Doctor about Your Tests

Question	Answer
What am I being tested for?	
Why do I need this test?	
When will the test be complete?	
How safe or risky is this test?	
How necessary is this test?	
Is the test routine?	
Is there an alternative to testing?	
Is there extra billing for the tests?	

5. Being Referred to a Specialist

When your GP sends you to a specialist, it is usually to request an opinion because the problem may be beyond the GP's scope of care. When this occurs you should ask the GP the reason for the referral.

Many people forget to ask any questions, especially if there is a concern of serious illness. They are often preoccupied with the possibility of a life-threatening illness.

Years of working in the mines had left Will, a husband and father of six children, with a hacking cough. When he was told that there was a possibility he had lung disease, the first thing that went through his mind was, "Who is going to look after my kids?" He wandered around for hours before going home, and it took him a few more hours before he could tell Cindy, his wife. She accompanied him on his visits to the doctor. She drew up a list of questions to ask, and when Will was too scared to even look the doctor in the eye, Cindy asked the questions and then repeated the answers to Will, to make sure he understood. See Checklist 15.

Checklist 15
What to Ask the Specialist

Question	Answer
When will you have the test results back?	
How will I know if there is a serious problem?	
Will you call us as soon as the x-rays results are in, or should I call you?	
What can you tell me about the seriousness of the condition?	
What can I expect of the medical resources offered by the doctors and community services?	
Will the follow-up visits be with the GP or with you?	

Each question touched on specific areas of concern to Will and Cindy. For example, once the specialist had diagnosed Will's condition, the specialist would oversee only relevant issues associated with the disease itself. The GP would then follow up with Will's ongoing care and treat any other ailments not associated with the disease. In this case, Will's condition turned out to be a bad lung infection rather than lung disease, which was treatable with an aggressive drug treatment plan.

6. What to Do When a Health-care Crisis Happens

When entering an emergency department, remember there are different degrees of health care needs. For instance, if persons arriving have been in a severe car accident, then the urgency of care is at a very different level of urgency than the person arriving with a broken leg. If some of the accident victims were unable to respond or give details about themselves at the time, then they are unable to convey details of the intensity of the injury so the physician must decipher this. However, the accident victims who are able to speak, including the person with a broken leg, can give the personal information needed before being seen by a doctor.

What to tell the doctor in an emergency:

- Tell a brief account of your medical history to the intake nurse or doctor.

- Tell the nurse or doctor what drugs you are taking.

- Tell the intake receptionist the name of a family member or friend.

- Tell the doctor where the pain or discomfort is located and its degree of intensity.

- Tell the nurse or doctor who your health-insurance provider is or about any extended health-insurance benefits.

- Tell the intake receptionist the name of your GP.

Remember, whether you are there on your own or on behalf of someone else, try to remain rational, calm, concise, clear, and informative.

Even though Sam seemed calm to Reba, when he had arrived at the emergency department with his wife he was panicky. She was having strong labor contractions. Because it was important to determine whether the mother or baby were in any danger, the doctors examined Aileen before collecting all her personal information. It turned out everything was normal and Aileen still had some time to go. With his wife settled on a gurney in the hallway, Sam sat down with the nurse and gave her specific details about his wife.

The nurse asked Sam the following questions:

- What is your wife's name?

- What is her birth date?

- What is her address?

- Do you have her health-insurance card available?

- Does she have extended health-insurance benefits?

- Who is her GP?

- What is her medical history, such as drugs or allergies?

- What drugs is she taking?

- What is her blood type?

- Is she an organ donor?

- How far apart are the contractions?

Most of these questions are part of the standard intake procedure in a hospital setting. Generally this interaction can be done calmly. However, when a health-care crisis happens, you have to act quickly. Be prepared to ask questions and tell accurate details about the crisis to a health-care provider.

Remember, the nature of the crisis and whether you are the patient or companion will influence how you proceed and what you say. Situations vary, and questions and the speediness of the process differ. Someone with a broken leg is not going to get attention as quickly someone having chest pains.

7. Chronic Health Problems

As we've seen, when someone is first diagnosed with an illness, it's often hard to seek information about the side effects or prognosis right away. News of a chronic illness can fuel a wide range of behavior such as denial, anger, bargaining, and sadness, which are emotions commonly associated with grief and dealing with death.

The following are the five steps of the grief process:

1. Denial of the symptoms of a chronic illness.

2. Anger in response to feelings of helplessness and futility because there are no answers to eliminating the inevitable ongoing illness.

3. Bargaining with God or promising to right the wrongs in one's life if the chronic illness can be reversed.

4. Sadness in response to letting go of the past.

5. Acceptance and resolution as a result of peace with the condition and finding other ways to move on.

These stages of grief generally, but not always, come in this order. Often depression is a side effect of such emotional impacts. Someone who is depressed hardly feels like seeking additional information or support groups. Feelings of anger and sadness sometimes affect the ability to listen or reach out to others. Sometimes we flounder until we meet with acceptance, but it is at this point that we usually surrender to our feelings. If we allow ourselves to feel those feelings instead of denying or minimizing them, we can move forward into a better future.

Often, actively trying to understand the why and what of an illness provides energy to battle the blows from such harsh realities of a chronic condition. Anger or panic often stimulates the energy required to search for information. That information gives you a base of knowledge, so you can interact with the doctor as an active participant, rather than a passive receiver. Even if you prefer to rely strictly on the facts given by the doctor, you will probably want to know something about recent research related to your condition.

8. Understanding Illness

The process of researching the details of an illness can be overwhelming. The physical and the mental drain of illness can be enough in itself. Nevertheless, such a search increases your knowledge about yourself and your situation. With information about symptoms, a chemical imbalance, chronic or terminal illness, and possible treatments, you can be an active participant in your health care.

If you want to understand your illness or that of someone close to you, there are approaches to researching the subject. (See Checklist 16.)

For instance, try setting aside one hour a day to read about it, either at home or at the library. The library provides a number of sources of information and librarians can be very helpful in identifying sources of medical information in books or on the Internet. They often know where to go for reliable websites and discussion groups.

If you have children at home, consider asking a friend or relative to babysit in exchange for your help on another occasion. Sometimes this is a welcome exchange, especially for mothers wanting a break. If you work, talk to colleagues who might know of helpful information resources. They might offer to find you information on the Internet. Browse in a bookstore for recent books. Ask your pharmacist and doctor for any materials related to your search; some keep information DVDs, lists, or handouts for providing information for patients. Once you have gathered the information, sort the facts from opinion and analyze and condense the facts into a list or a small report for quick reference.

Many chronic and life-threatening diseases have sparked support and research organizations. For example, Breast Cancer Action has centers across North America that invite speakers to address varying aspects of the disease. Often these speakers are breast cancer survivors. Just listening to them might offer you the support you need.

Most local community clinics and hospitals have a library room and provide counseling services for anyone. Nonprofit organizations, such as the Heart and Stroke Foundation, Multiple Sclerosis Society, Mental Health Association, and Schizophrenia Society, are also good sources of information and support, and most have their own websites. (See the Resources at the end of this book or in the download kit.)

Check your local bookstore or library for reference books with updated listings of websites. Always take care to verify the validity of some of the information provided: Check for evidence-based research by health-care practitioners or researchers. In other words, is the medical information and advice you find certified by medical practitioners?

9. Building a Support Network

During the progression of any illness, whether you are the person who is sick or that person's caregiver, a good communication network with others helps keep a link to the outside world at a time when it may be all too easy to retreat. Reaching out for support from a close friend or relative, volunteer, counselor, or spiritual advisor can enhance your ability to remain positive and help you accept your position as patient or caregiver. Your doctor or community health center usually has a variety of information and resources specific to your condition.

Checklist 16
Ask the Doctor

Question	Answer
Can you give me any reference materials on my condition?	
Will you help me decide on the best approach?	
Will you give me occasional direction and support as my condition progresses?	
When should I follow up with you?	
Would drug therapy combined with counseling help?	

For one reason or another you might prefer to look for a support group on your own. You can start by the standard methods of looking for listings in the telephone book, Yellow Pages, library, and classified advertisements in the newspaper. By using the Internet, you have access to a wide range of information, such as personal support groups and chat groups. Search engines such as Yahoo! and Google among others list innumerable support group sites for almost every disease or illness. Local health clinics, hospitals, community centers, and other community-based groups often have many ongoing personal support groups.

Jill's doctor told her she should slow down her fast-paced lifestyle to avoid becoming ill from stress. At this point her symptoms included mild bowel irritability, back pain, and tension headaches — too many to ignore.

Her doctor gave her information pamphlets that described different approaches and resource groups. Jill then discussed their success rate with her doctor. Together they agreed on a six-week group program for stress management in a hospital setting. They also agreed that going swimming once a week and one night of weekly entertainment would help lead to a healthier lifestyle.

9.1 Personal support groups

Support groups might be located close at hand; however, many people, especially those living in rural areas, might have to travel to meet with a group. If any members of the group live near you, you could carpool. Consider developing a buddy system in which one or two people can give you support over the telephone or via email, you might want to start your own support group close to home.

Bella, recently informed she had a chronic autoimmune condition, was exhausted by its effects on her neuromuscular system. Its long-term effects weakened her muscles, and her lungs, adding to her physical and mental exhaustion.

As with many chronic diseases, Bella felt alone with the symptoms until she discovered others diagnosed with the same condition. Her doctor had given her the names of two support groups operating in the local hospital and a community health clinic. Bella also went to some seminars offered at the hospital. Most of what she heard about her condition was already familiar to her from her own research. At the support groups, the discussions tended to focus on the negative aspects of the illness, without discussing the positive and management sides. She wanted to learn more about how to manage the disease instead of dwelling on what she could not change. She went back to her GP to discuss the problem.

"Doctor, I really don't get anything from those support groups. They're always talking about what's wrong," said Bella. "I'd rather focus on how to better manage the symptoms."

"I understand," replied the doctor. "Is there anyone in either of the groups who feels the same way you do?"

"As a matter of fact, yes," said Bella. "They are a couple of people."

"Perhaps you could speak with them about how you feel and see if you can discuss this openly at the next meeting," suggested the doctor.

"Why don't you take the lead? It sounds like a shift in focus would improve the benefits of the group atmosphere."

"That's a good idea, but maybe those two people would come over to my place," said Bella. "We could help each other on managing the symptoms."

"You could try that too," said the doctor. "Suggest it to them at your next meeting, or call them if you've got their phone numbers. Don't forget to tell the group leader about your decision."

Bella and two other women decided to start meeting once a week to discuss coping strategies. The subject of discomfort only arose in the context of how those strategies were working. Each member brought new ideas to share with the others.

Each week they had an agenda and primary focus for the first hour. Each person talked of progress or setbacks, with a group discussion and support for succeeding or struggling with managing the symptoms. The rest of their gathering shifted to social interaction with coffee and snacks. Soon they began to meet once a month instead of weekly, and rotated the location of the meeting among the three members' homes.

Ask your doctor for more detailed information or where to look for reliable information on a specific condition. Ask your pharmacist. Consult the local librarian, and search your Government Health websites. Ask people at community health clinics or health-related nonprofit organizations. Many of these places have books, CDs, and DVDs full of information.

You will find a number of helpful volunteers or paid workers to guide you once you have made contact with some of these resources. Often these people can lead you to additional references. Speaking with friends or relatives also produces surprisingly positive support.

You can verify the information you find with a doctor you respect, especially if you're trying to understand the meaning behind medical terminology, side effects, prognosis, or long-term effects. The doctor can also offer moral support and crucial insights into coping with illness.

Another benefit of asking the doctor for information is that you get an indication of how much the doctor knows about your condition. For example, a doctor might not feel comfortable treating a patient with an eating disorder. Most doctors in this situation would refer the patient to another doctor, but if you sense that your doctor is uncomfortable, discuss this with your doctor, or ask for a referral.

Remember: You and your doctor must feel comfortable with each other when asking questions or discussing treatment plans. Your doctor must be able to keep you informed or guide you in learning about the diagnosis and prognosis of your condition.

Your role is to absorb the information, question, learn, and work toward recovery or toward coping with a variety of feelings. In part, this involves having a sense of what is best for you. Everyone's needs vary and that sometimes means working through the initial emotional upheaval alone. Most of us need to take an active approach to find out what information can be helpful in a time of crisis. You decide what is your preference.

10. When Doctors Have No Answers

We don't want to think that there is no answer to what ails us. However, the reality is that health-care professionals do not always have the answers. This is as frustrating for them as it is for you. The doctor might have to resort to giving you innumerable painkillers or other medications thought to minimize symptom effects, and you might keep visiting the doctor for recurring discomfort. You might even resist accepting the fact that there is no miracle cure or one pill to alleviate your pain. Letting go of this idea requires a lot of re-evaluation of yourself and the situation, and possibly changing your attitude and lifestyle.

Judy's doctor, although supportive, told her after a few months of treating her for chronic pain that there was no answer to eliminating the pain. All he could do was give her painkillers. He encouraged her to consider a combination of physiotherapy, diet changes, and anti-inflammatory pills that would help her manage the pain. Although at first she was depressed by the prospect of living with pain, she eventually accepted that there were options other than drug therapy. Judy went on to develop her own pain management program, which relied heavily on nondrug therapy.

11. When You Should Get a Second Opinion

Many of you have probably contemplated getting another opinion for one reason or another. Maybe you didn't go through with it because you were not sure it was appropriate to do so. You need to get another opinion when the following occurs:

- You are unsure of the doctor's diagnosis.

- You don't trust the doctor.

- Your insurance company requires you to have a second opinion.

- The diagnosis is serious.

- The recommended treatment is extreme.

- You are uncomfortable about the appropriateness of a doctor's behavior.

- You are considering recommended surgery.

- You cannot get the doctor to communicate in a way that you understand.

As for figuring out how to find someone for a second opinion, finding a doctor is the subject of the next chapter.

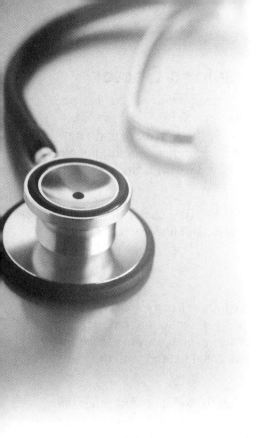

7

Searching for a New Doctor

Finding a new doctor involves a number of steps. First you need to consider why you need a new doctor. Then you need to begin a broad search, contacting one or two doctor referral services, talking to friends, and tapping into other information resources. After you gather names of doctors taking new patients, you need to interview the doctors. Based on your impressions of those interviews, you will likely be able to make a final choice for a doctor.

Reasons to look for a new GP:

- Your GP is retiring, moving, or closing the practice.

- You are a new resident in the area.

- Your GP has behaved inappropriately or unprofessionally.

- You have difficulty communicating with your GP.

- You and your GP have philosophically different approaches to health care.

1. Approaches to Looking for a Doctor

Usually a GP who decides to close a practice provides his or her patients with the names of several other doctors. Some people are satisfied taking their GP's recommendation, and others prefer to find a new doctor on their own. Let's take a look at the experience of five people who shared the same doctor and how they dealt with the news that their GP was moving to another city.

The following sections discuss how Karey, Lee, Alfred, Devon, and Chelsea proceeded in their search, interview, and final choice of a new doctor.

1.1 Be prepared

Karey is a single woman in her 30s who works as a marketing coordinator. For her, the doctor's gender and age were important criteria. She thought that a female doctor close to her own age would make for easier interaction with the doctor. She decided to start with the three names her GP referred her to.

Karey set aside some time one evening to work out what other criteria were important and to prepare for interviewing the prospective choices. She developed the following list of questions for evaluating the doctor's compatibility with her:

- Does the doctor have a caring personality?

- Does the doctor's interaction style feel comfortable to me?

- Does the doctor listen to me?

- Is the doctor sympathetic toward my lifestyle?

- Is the doctor willing to negotiate differences of opinion?

- Does the doctor stay up to date on medical research?

- Does the doctor plan to stay in the area for some time?

- Do we have similar views on methods of treatment?

- Is the doctor available in emergency situations?

- Does the doctor respect my wishes with regard to life and death situations?

Once she had written this list, Karey thought about how she could shape the content of these questions into a reasonable interview format, without putting the doctor on the defensive. To help her, she asked a friend for feedback. Eventually, she worked out something that felt comfortable to her. This is how one of her interviews went:

Karey was waiting in the doctor's office when the doctor arrived. "Hi," said the doctor in a friendly tone. "How are you today?"

"Fine thanks," replied Karey, although she was a little nervous. "I'm looking for a new doctor, and my current GP gave me your name."

"Yes, I understand he is retiring."

"Yes, that's right," replied Karey. "I'm trying to make up my mind about a few things before I make a decision. Do you mind if I ask you a few questions?"

"No, I don't mind at all," answered the doctor. "What would you like to know?"

"Could we first talk about what you might suggest about some of my health concerns? Oh, and — " she looked at her notes, "I wondered if you are planning to keep your practice here?"

"Yes," said the doctor with a smile. "I expect to stay in this area for some time. Of course, sometimes this kind of thing is hard to predict. But my practice is well established and I like it here. As for suggestions, perhaps you could give me an idea of what concerns you have."

"I'm not thinking of anything specific," said Karey. "I want to get an idea of what kind of approaches you take."

"I'm inclined toward following the usual medical conventions, but I'm open to discussing alternatives," said the doctor. "Of course, a lot depends on the particular problem needing treatment, but I find that there are many different approaches to consider."

"I'm glad to hear that, because I'm more comfortable with conventional medicine but I'm kind of curious about herbal medicines," said Karey.

"I understand," the doctor said. "Is there anything else you would like to ask me?"

"I have a busy schedule and sometimes I am called away unexpectedly to attend a business meeting. What if I had an appointment with you and I had to cancel at the last minute — would I be charged for the missed appointment?"

"No, I don't bill if it's an emergency situation out of your control," said the doctor. "I'd appreciate, though, if you could try to call ahead of time whenever possible."

"Of course," said Karey. As she went on with her questions, she discovered that the doctor met her expectations. She also felt comfortable with the doctor's friendly manner and treatment approaches, and their courteous and casual conversation helped to create a relaxed atmosphere. For these reasons, she decided immediately that she would like this doctor to oversee any future health concerns.

1.2 Use a positive approach

Lee is a single, 20-year-old college student with an interest in recreational athletics. He occasionally has sports injuries. The doctor's gender or age did not matter to Lee as long as the doctor was familiar with sports injuries and the chronic pain they sometimes cause. He also wrote a list of questions to ask, but did not bother to prepare himself for interviewing the doctor, and forgot the list when he met with the doctor. His conversation with a male doctor was very different than Karey's.

"Hi," said the doctor. "What can I do for you today?"

"Didn't my other doctor tell you why I was coming to see you?" said Lee testily. "I thought he was going to!"

"Yes, he did call me," said the doctor. "You seem a bit upset. Are you upset with your doctor leaving?"

Lee slouched back in the chair. "It doesn't make much difference to me," he said. "I don't go to the doctor much anyway."

"So when do you feel it is necessary to see a doctor?"

Lee suddenly remembered why he was there. "I kind of wanted to ask you a few questions about how you work."

"What did you have in mind?" The doctor was surprised by Lee's abrupt change of topic.

"What's your specialty anyway?" asked Lee. "What if there's an emergency, do I have to go to the hospital or what? I need a doctor who knows about sports injuries; you've got to know something about sports."

Lee's evasive and aggressive manner set a negative tone during the meeting. His challenging approach placed the doctor on the defensive, leaving little room for a potentially positive patient-doctor relationship. Lee was not allowing himself any opportunity to find out if he and the doctor were a good fit. How could he have handled this interaction differently?

Instead of reacting to the doctor, Lee could have immediately introduced his reason for wanting to find a new doctor. That would be a good time to mention that he did not make frequent visits. He could also have expressed his preference for a doctor familiar with treating sports injuries. By stating these facts, he would have created a different atmosphere, and would have gotten answers to any questions he might have had. The conversation could have gone like this:

Lee could have opened with "Hi, thank you for seeing me."

"It's nice to meet you," the doctor might have responded. "I understand that you are looking for a new doctor. Are there any questions you would like to ask me?"

"Yes, I wonder if you treat many people with sport injuries. I have chronic pain in my shoulder from playing hockey. What would you recommend for the pain? I also had a few other questions, but I left my list at home and I've forgotten most of them. Maybe you can help me. I'm not sure of what I should be asking in a first visit."

The doctor would likely respond favorably to this kind of approach. He might prompt Lee's memory by asking him when and why he might feel a need to visit the doctor. Then Lee would be able to say that he usually only consults a doctor when he has a sports injury. The doctor, who in this case also had an interest in sport activities, could use this common interest as a point of discussion, thus allowing for an easier conversation.

1.3 Find someone you're comfortable with seeing

Alfred is a happily retired widower who spends much of his time playing bridge and golf. He wanted a middle-aged doctor who would be around for another 20 years, because that's at least how long he expected to live.

Of the three names his former GP gave him one was a doctor about 20 years younger than Alfred. Alfred didn't think it necessary to write a list of questions. His only concern was whether the doctor "planned to live as long as he did." When he asked the doctor this question, the doctor laughed. "It's certainly in my immediate plans," he said. Alfred was satisfied with the interaction and chose this doctor as his primary health-care provider.

1.4 Decide what is important for you

An engineer by profession, Devon is 40 and divorced. He was not sure what he was looking for since he rarely visited the doctor. He thought he would prefer a recent medical graduate setting up a new practice because he figured that this would place him in the hands of someone with knowledge of the latest medical research and health-care approaches.

Devon met with all three of the doctors recommended by his former doctor. None of these doctors seemed to satisfy him. When he discussed this with a friend, they talked about questions Devon could ask the doctors. His friend suggested Devon take some time to decide what was important to him.

Devon asked himself a set of questions to help him in his search:

- Is the doctor's communication style important to me?

- Are the doctor's knowledge and interest in alternative medicine important to me?

- Is it important that the doctor is open to making final decisions for my health care?

- Is the doctor's openness to joint decision making for my health care important to me?

- Is having the doctor's office near my home important?

When he considered the answers to these questions, only the last one was unimportant to him. He determined what key points were significant, and then started looking for new doctors.

Devon began by calling the doctor referral services of the Royal College of Physicians and Surgeons, and the College of Family Physicians for a list of doctors in his area who were taking new patients. He added a couple of names of doctors from the community health clinic. He made a point of asking the people who supplied the names for any specifics about the doctor's reputation, personal manner, and style. When he was through he had the names of three doctors.

As he prepared to interview them, he kept his questions similar to his original list. He started with a male doctor, whose age was about the same as his own.

"How are you today?" asked the doctor.

"Very good, thank you," said Devon. "I'm looking for a new doctor and wondered if I could ask you a few questions."

"What exactly do you want to know?" asked the doctor a little defensively. The interview with this doctor continued to be tense. Based on this feeling, Devon moved on to the next doctor.

The next doctor was female and within his age range.

"Hello, how are you today?" she asked.

"Fine thanks," replied Devon.

"I'm looking for a new doctor because my former doctor is retiring. I have chosen three doctors to talk to about a few things I feel are important. Do you mind if I ask you a few questions? "

"Sure, no problem," answered the doctor. "What would you like to know?"

Devon began asking his questions, including what she would recommend for the pain he occasionally felt in his left shoulder. She answered all of his questions in a pleasant and honest manner, and she did not appear at all rushed. Devon was pleased with how the interview went; nevertheless, he went on to interview the last doctor on his referral list. She was also female, and was about ten years his senior.

"What can I do for you today?" Her manner was cold and business-like.

"Well, I'm looking for a new doctor and — "

"So my receptionist tells me," interrupted the doctor. "You wanted to interview me?"

"Yes, I planned to ask you a few questions about your approach to health care."

"If what you're asking is do I use alternative medicine, the answer is no," she said. "I'm not interested in that nonsense. I stick to what's proven and works."

Devon quickly decided not to continue with the rest of the questions. He politely thanked her for her time and excused himself.

Devon made a final decision. He chose the second doctor, who had 15 years' experience. He felt he could talk with her easily. He called her office to make an appointment for a regular checkup, and then, as a courtesy, he left follow-up messages with the other two doctors to let them know he would not be seeing them.

1.5 Similar views on treatment

Chelsea is a 35-year-old lawyer and single mother. She wanted a female, middle-aged GP with a progressive attitude, who was open to homeopathy as well as conventional approaches to medicines, to provide care for herself and her son, who has a hip deformity that causes him to limp. She preferred someone open to joint decision making. She also wanted a doctor with a wide variety of patients. Her present doctor was only able to refer her to one doctor, who did not have certification in homeopathy, so she started her own search.

First she prepared two sets of questions to form a basis for interviewing a doctor. The first half of questions related to the doctor's patient load and the second half related to health-care treatments:

- What are the demographics of the doctor's patient load?

- What percentage of patients are children?

- What percentage of patients are seniors or aging?

- What percentage of patients are chronically ill?

- What percentage of patients have physical or mental disabilities?

- How culturally diverse are the patients as a group?

- How economically diverse are the patients as a group?

- What are the doctor's criteria for choosing one approach over another?

- What medical approach would you recommend if my child had a slight fever?

- What annual vaccinations do you recommend for my child, if any?

- What objections would you have if I preferred my child not be vaccinated?

- What do you know about my child's disability?

- What are the long-term effects on his overall health?

- What approach would you recommend if I had a persistent heavy cough?

- What do you recommend for stress relief?

Her list provided for her some idea of the balance of medical approaches and treatments the doctor might recommend in varying circumstances.

With her list of questions in hand, Chelsea searched the pages of the telephone book for doctors' names. She contacted the local school of homeopathy to check the required training for homeopathic practitioners; they gave her general information about the different schools of thought on homeopathic methodology.

In her conversations with the people at a community health clinic she was given the name of a medically trained doctor who had seven years' apprenticeship in homeopathy. She decided to interview that doctor too.

"Hi," said the doctor. "How are you today?"

"I feel fine today," said Chelsea. "I do have migraines on occasion, but that's not why I'm here today. My GP is moving his practice, so I need to find a new doctor."

"I see," said the doctor. "Would you like to ask me any questions?"

Chelsea was pleased that the doctor asked her this question. It saved her from having to introduce the idea. "As a matter of fact," she said, "I have a list of questions. May I show you the list and then we could discuss them?"

"Of course," said the doctor. "Let's have a look." He read the list quickly. "I see you have questions here about my views on homeopathy as well as conventional medical treatments."

"Yes, I think homeopathic treatments could be well suited for some things. But I know conventional medicine has a lot to offer. What's your training?"

"I have a medical degree from an accredited school," said the doctor, "and I am a certified homeopath. Can you give me an example of what kind of problem you would want treated?"

"How about those migraines I mentioned?"

"First," said the doctor, "I would take an overall history of your health, including your emotional responses to life challenges. Then I would ask the nature of the migraines, how long you've had them, and what you've been using to decrease the pain."

"Then what?" asked Chelsea. "Would you recommend a homeopathic approach first or conventional medicine?"

"I would go over the complete report with you, make recommendations for both approaches, and then we would try to reach a common decision."

"This sounds good to me," said Chelsea, smiling. "Now, what if I didn't want to go along with your suggestions?"

"Do you mean what if you presented a different approach?"

Chelsea nodded.

"As long as it did not endanger your health, I would encourage your final decision. However, if you continued to have problems, I'd probably try to persuade you to try my suggestions."

"I like that."

Chelsea had arrived at a number of conclusions from her meeting with the doctor. She recognized that the doctor was open to negotiating with her. She also noted that the doctor had Chelsea's best interest at heart in terms of taking control of the situation if Chelsea's choices were dangerous to her health or her son's. She liked the doctor's openness and knowledge in both areas of health treatment. Chelsea also discovered that the doctor encouraged a practical approach to keeping well through exercise and eating a balanced diet. She had no difficulty making the final decision to become this doctor's patient. Chelsea's easy-going interview approach kept the meeting relaxed and oriented to her needs.

1.6 Good communication is important

Karey, Lee, Devon, Alfred, and Chelsea each considered how their needs would be met by assessing each doctor's personal and professional manner. Each preferred doctors who communicated freely and displayed understanding, knowledge, trust, and openness. To achieve a successful exchange with the doctor, they realized that they too had to communicate. By determining which doctor they could achieve this level of exchange with meant deciding what they wanted in a doctor.

Each person followed more or less the same process. First they listed questions to help them decide what they were looking for in a doctor. That list set the stage for the search and helped them ask concise questions. Then they evaluated the doctors' responses to their questions and, after assessing their personal impressions, made a final decision. Each took responsibility for his or her role in the patient-doctor relationship, which will ultimately contribute to better health care for them.

In the process, Karey, Lee, Devon, Alfred, and Chelsea each concluded that developing a trust in their doctor's ability to treat them depended on a gut feeling and their later experience with the doctor. Apart from liking and trusting the doctor, these patients also trusted their own instincts as to what felt good for them.

If you are looking for a new doctor, you'll have your own personal style and approach to researching, interviewing, and making a final decision. The criteria you choose will influence the time and energy you spend at the various stages. Of course, other considerations, such as your age and health, influence the type of questions you ask and which doctor you choose to advise you on health care.

Checklist 17
Questions to Ask a Potential New Doctor

The following questions are considerations to keep in mind when choosing a new doctor. Not every question will apply to your situation.

Question	Answer
Does the doctor seem to have a caring personality?	
Does the doctor's interaction style feel comfortable to me?	
Does the doctor listen to me?	
Is the doctor sympathetic toward my lifestyle?	
Is the doctor willing to negotiate differences of opinion?	
Does the doctor stay up to date on medical research?	
Does the doctor plan to stay in the area for some time?	
Do we have similar views on methods of treatment?	
Is the doctor available in emergency situations?	
Does the doctor respect my wishes with regard to life and death situations?	
Does the doctor have knowledge and interest in alternative medicine?	
Is the doctor open to making final decisions for my health care?	
Is the doctor open to joint decision making for my health care?	
What are the doctor's criteria for choosing one approach over another?	
What percentage of patients are seniors or aging?	

What percentage of patients are chronically ill?	
What percentage of patients have physical or mental disabilities?	
What percentage of patients are children?	
What medical approach would you recommend if my child had a slight fever?	
What annual vaccinations do you recommend for my child, if any?	
What objections would you have if I preferred my child not be vaccinated?	
What do you know about my child's disability?	
What approach would you recommend if I had a persistent heavy cough?	
What do you recommend for stress relief?	
After the interview, you may want to ask yourself the following questions:	
Did the doctor listen to what I said?	
Did I feel comfortable with the doctor's personality?	
Am I comfortable with the doctor's communication style?	
Does the doctor share my views on health-care approaches?	
Am I interested in listening to what the doctor says?	

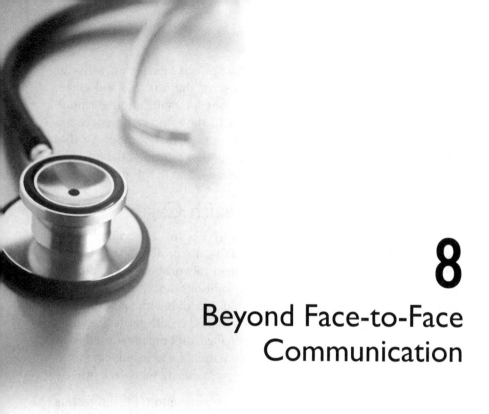

8

Beyond Face-to-Face Communication

It's my hope that in the process of reading this book you have had time to reflect on some of the stories, along with the communication strategies used in the various situations. My hope also is that you have learned from these people's experiences and learned to adapt your own communication style to improve your interactions with your doctor.

Now you can evaluate how you interpret what your doctor says. You can comfortably express how you feel physically and emotionally. With the skills described in this book, you're ahead of all those who assume that what we understand and what we say are only expressed through speaking. After all, as you know, there is more to the communication process than just words. As you speak, you use your voice like an instrument to produce many sounds and inflections. You use your ears to receive simple or complex words, hoping that you understand what is being said. You increase your understanding of what is said by listening attentively. Using knowledge like this will lead you to better health care.

However, as you continue to communicate with your doctor you need to be aware of technological advances in communication and how technology will continue to be part of our interaction with our health-care providers. The expanding use of the Internet and email, along with teleconferencing (i.e., using telecommunications technology to link participants in different sites to the same conference) and telemedicine (i.e., using telecommunications/virtual technology that enables doctors to diagnose and treat patients from separate locations) provide hints of how quickly we are moving in this direction.

1. Internet, Email, and Health Care

By using the Internet, people can have access to health information that was once only accessible to health-care professionals. Consequently, many people have developed medical vocabularies that bring them closer to understanding medical conditions described by doctors. Because of the increased use of technology with health care, the relationship between you and the doctor or allied health professionals is changing. Continued use of virtual medicine (sometimes referred to as interactive technology) is changing how patients and health-care practitioners view each other and how we communicate with each other.

As time passes, you will probably become comfortable interacting with health-care professionals through interactive technology, just as you have in using automatic bank machines. Medical terminology will become second nature when we speak about sickness, wellness, and health care. We already often act as information gatherers of recent research on various diseases and chronic illnesses, passing condensed versions of this information on to our doctors.

Granted, some people will always prefer the traditional face-to-face patient-doctor interaction. Some, however, will embrace the use of virtual medicine or interactive technology, such as those already mentioned. The latter telecommunications, still relatively new in the health-care system, will intrigue some enough that they will want to learn more about its future place in our lives.

2. Interacting with Doctors in the Future

The current uses of the Internet and email are going to expand as we move into the future. Virtual medicine or telecommunication will be used more and more to transmit patient and medical information. We will be expected to communicate more often by using email, interactive video, and teleconferencing. Already some GPs and specialists communicate with one another using new technology, whether they're on the other side of the world or just across town.

Although these practices are not yet widespread, doctors can already monitor the blood sugar (or glucose) of someone with diabetes through electronic links that transmit the information from the person at home to the doctor in the office. The person places one finger in a clip, which is plugged into an electronic device that allows the blood sugar levels to be measured, giving the doctor information needed to make any changes in insulin therapy.

2.1 What is telemedicine?

Telemedicine, sometimes referred to as telehealth, is the present and future of our health care. As explained above, it is an electronic link between a patient and a doctor who can be far apart, and involves technologies such as distance education and video conferencing to deliver pictures and sound. It also allows GPs, specialists, and allied health professionals to consult using a computer monitor. Telemedicine saves time, money, and lives, and makes possible speedier diagnoses and recovery for people in remote locations.

Since around 1994, hospitals have been working on telemedicine projects, sometimes coordinated by allied health professionals. By definition, a doctor's telephone consultation is a form of telemedicine, but with the sophisticated new technology now becoming available, new dimensions will be added to how we communicate with our doctors.

Ron explored some of these new dimensions further when he and his girlfriend Marta visited TJ and Francine. They discussed some of the effects of new technology over dinner.

"When my GP calls me back," said Ron, "we communicate differently than if we were face to face. We listen more intently to our words and provide more explanation because there isn't any body language to accent our words."

"That's right, Ron," said Marta. "And email adds a whole other dimension to the way you communicate with your doctor."

"What do you mean?" asked Francine.

"Picture this," said Marta. "Ron sends his doctor an email that says: Hi, doctor, I have a question for you about something I read on the

Internet. This guy in a chat group on supplements says that if I take mega-vitamins it will increase my energy level. It's been low lately. What do you think? Signed, Ron."

"I think the doctor would probably ask Ron for more details, just like he would in person," said TJ. "He'd need to know who the person is giving the advice."

"Right," said Ron. "He'd want to know if the sender is an MD or a naturopath or maybe a nutritionist, and what kind of credentials he has, or a scammer. The same kind of information I should be watching out for!"

"He'd want to know more details about Ron's symptoms," said Marta. "He'd probably suggest he make an appointment and bring in a copy of the correspondence, or maybe ask Ron to forward it to him, so they could tackle the issue of Ron's energy problem."

"I can see why some doctors might like this email business," said Francine. "If their patients keep the channels of communication open like that, then they can monitor the kind of information their patients are receiving."

"Yes," said Ron. "Don't you think a doctor who's open to email correspondence would probably be up to date in other areas too, and open to new ideas?"

"Oh yes, probably," said Marta.

"Wait a minute," TJ said. "The doctor would still expect you to provide details by email, the same as if you were to visit your doctor in person. The only difference is that you need to be more detailed in your written communication, right?"

"Yes, of course that's part of it," said Marta. "Patients need to be able to clearly organize their thoughts in writing, which as we know is not always easy for some people. Right, Ron?"

"I'm sure I don't know what you're talking about," chuckled Ron.

"Don't you work in a hospital, Marta?" asked Francine.

"Yes. In fact, that's how I met Ron. He called looking to speak to someone about telemedicine. I'm the nurse-coordinator of our telemedicine pilot project."

"That explains Ron's sudden interest in the health-care system," said TJ.

Marta smiled. "Actually, there's a lot to learn," she said. "I'm still on a learning curve myself. It's fascinating stuff."

"What is telemedicine or what some people call virtual medicine, anyway?" asked Francine.

"Marta will correct me if I'm wrong, but let's say for example you live in a remote town quite some distance from any city," said Ron. "You have two small kids, and you can't get into town easily. You also have some kind of a chronic condition that needs to be monitored by your GP. If you can afford it, you'd use your computer and set up some kind of Skype conferencing system to allow you to talk with your doctor about how you're doing."

"Right," said Marta. "You'd save a lot of time of traveling back and forth into the city."

"What do you mean, 'if you can afford it'?" asked TJ. "What if you can't afford it?"

"This is part of the program that's still being worked out," said Ron. "I'm not sure of all the details. Are you, Marta?"

"Some rural hospitals are setting up telemedicine programs to provide access to the health-care services that aren't available in that community."

"I imagine that at some point there'll be community health centers in small towns with similar access, too," said Ron. "There are certainly glitches in the system that have to be smoothed out."

"Yes," said Marta. "We still have a way to go before this becomes common practice, although you're right about there being support for it in remote areas, especially in places like Alaska or in the remote parts of Quebec or Yukon. You know, places that are hard to reach."

"Makes sense, I guess the further away, the more it is needed." said Francine.

"Yes," said Ron. "People also have to get used to the idea. Marta, remember the story of that man who demanded telemedicine?"

Marta smiled. "Oh yes, that was so funny. We had an elderly gentleman with heart problems who told the doctor that he wanted telemedicine. I don't know where he'd heard about it, but he didn't really understand it. When the doctor said she wasn't involved in telemedicine, he said, 'Get me a doctor who can give me some! I want telemedicine!'"

Marta pounded the table as she spoke, as the others started to laugh. "The doctor had quite a time trying to explain to the man that telemedicine isn't a little pill."

"Can't you just imagine the poor guy scratching his head, trying to figure it all out?" asked TJ.

"Yes," said Ron. "I guess people hear about it on TV or read about it in the paper. Anyway, the GP has to do most of the communicating for the patient, and a lot depends on the seriousness of the patient's condition. It would be possible for the patient to consult with the GP and the specialist all at the same time through telemedicine."

"That's amazing," said TJ.

"It is!" said Ron. "Let's say the doctor has to consult a couple of specialists about a particular x-ray, but they're all in different hospitals in different cities or even a different country. They can interface about a patient's results as well as see the x-ray because of the system's computer-generated imaging. They can consult as a team and quickly transmit their diagnoses electronically, without having to fuss with travel time and meetings. The patient can be involved in the Skype conference too — if the patient is injured or something, the doctors can actually see the injury on their screens. It's so intriguing!" Ron paused to contemplate his thoughts, then went on to say, "Yep, that is why some call it virtual medicine."

Marta laughed at Ron's enthusiasm.

"Wait a minute," said TJ. "Do you mean that if the x-ray showed signs of heart disease the GP could get feedback from a specialist almost immediately?"

"Exactly. Well, not all. It depends if the GP has the updated technology in his or her office," said Marta. "However, last week we had a patient with symptoms of angina-heart pain and the patient was in one of the places where we've set up a pilot virtual medicine program. As soon as the cardiologist received the cardiogram and x-rays, a consultation time was set. The process of assessment took place with the patient at home and the doctor in the hospital."

"What kind of equipment do you need?" asked Francine.

"There's a platform or metal casing that contains a computer, a video screen, a video camera, and some other equipment. There's one platform at each end, so there's one at the patient's end, and another at each doctor's location. The camera allows the doctor to look at a screen at that location and see the patient at the remote site. The patient sees the doctor on a video or computer screen as well."

"Usually the first consultation is just an interview, right Marta?" asked Ron.

"Yes, that's right."

"How does the patient know how to use the equipment?" asked TJ.

"There are specially trained nurses at both ends who know how to make the equipment work for both parties. At the patient's end, the nurse usually provides chart information or other information to the doctor. The nurse acts as the doctor's hands and the doctor guides the nurse. So the nurse and the doctor do the assessment together."

"How does the doctor know if the nurse is giving accurate feedback?" asked Francine.

"That's part of the training; the nurse learns the skills required for assessment."

"It really seems odd in a way, don't you think?" asked TJ.

Ron laughed. "Like some kind of science fiction story, but it's really happening. I've seen a nurse use a special electronic stethoscope so the doctor can actually hear the patient's heart — the patient was in Alaska and the doctor was in Toronto! This can even work from one side of the world to another, for example from Japan to Boston."

"Is it very different from the doctor being right there, face to face?" asked Francine.

"Not really," said Marta, "because the doctor and patient can see and hear each other so the body language comes across. The doctor can see the patient's reactions."

"Hmmm," said Francine, "I just remembered a friend of mine in a small town in Oregon who told me about a support group experiment she participated in that involved audio teleconferencing. She was very impressed with the support she got from the group. Is audio teleconferencing part of telemedicine, Marta?"

"Yes, as a matter of fact it was developed at the telemedicine center at Memorial University in Newfoundland. "

"The more I learn about this subject, the more I want to explore," said Ron. "So they had a support group of people spread out all over the place who communicated by voice but not by video or by Skyping?"

"That's what my friend described," said Francine.

"It was a support group for people with breast cancer, wasn't it?" said Marta. "I know there are some starting up now in the field of psychiatry."

"It was the breast cancer one. My friend's cancer was recently diagnosed. One of the things she said worked really well about the group was that people could participate anonymously. They got the benefit of sharing their thoughts and experiences with people going through the same struggles as they were," said Francine. "My friend said it really lifted her feelings of being alone, even though there were people at all different stages of the disease."

2.2 Patients' response to telemedicine

Only a small percentage of patients are not interested in participating in telemedicine. Most people who have used telemedicine are comfortable with it, especially because it usually produces quicker solutions to their problems. The system has been carefully designed to protect patients' privacy and confidentiality, and the benefits outweigh the risks to privacy in most instances.

In addition to the benefits to patients, doctors in remote locations benefit from access to specialists and other resources. This improves their satisfaction with their rural practice so they are more likely to stay put, which is an issue of concern for many communities across North America.

Many of us have probably already observed examples of telemedicine without even knowing its name. This will change as broadcast, print, and electronic media educate the public. I am sure with the new technologies coming along that even more clarity and inventiveness will be developed to provide even better health care. I think we have only seen the tip of the iceberg as is said.

2.3 Occasional doctor resistance to telemedicine

Some doctors are reluctant to get involved in virtual or telemedicine because some of the health-care maintenance organization and plans have yet to decide which telemedicine services will be insured. Established guidelines for doctor's billing for services provided through email or Internet also are vague. Questions arise about licensing, jurisdictions, and payment (i.e., who pays for the service when a doctor in one city or country interprets an x-ray sent from a rural area in another location). Usually, the referring site pays for the service, but it is not always clear to the doctor or patient. These uncertainties can create valid concerns for those involved. With time, however, government insurance or health maintenance organization policies will hopefully have better established guidelines.

Some doctors might find offering consultations over the Internet or through teleconferencing more appealing if a fee-for-service arrangement is made possible through public or government funding. Most doctors, however, prefer consulting with a patient over the telephone rather than by email or the Internet. They find it less risky than treading on the unfamiliar ground of using new technology they do not yet understand.

Some doctors also feel reluctant to participate in virtual/telemedicine because the regulations that govern doctors do not yet offer legal protection when offering medical advice to a patient communicating from another country. The vague guidelines leave most doctors hesitant to offer medical advice over the Internet or email, especially to patients outside their jurisdiction. International guidelines of doctor accountability for medical advice differ from one country to another.

Some specialists fear that their services might not be needed anymore thanks to the use of telemedicine. For example, a specialist in a rural area might fear losing patients because local GPs will refer directly to a telemedicine clinic, bypassing the specialist.

However, most GPs in rural areas welcome the expediency that telemedicine has to offer. They can have a patient assessed more quickly and safely than if the patient is transported to the city.

Obviously, there are pros and cons for the medical community and the public. The biggest advantage is that virtual or telemedicine is sophisticated technology that benefits the doctor and the patient in ways that might not otherwise be possible. The disadvantages are that the technology is intimidating for some and not yet affordable for others.

In time, however, the glitches will be balanced by the benefits because of pressure from those in the medical community promoting the advantages of virtual or telemedicine to the patient population. You can expect that virtual/telemedicine will close the gap between rural and urban medicine, giving many North Americans better access to health care.

3. Closing the Communication Gap

The communication strategies suggested throughout this book concentrate on patient communication with GPs, in part because of the central role that GPs play in our health care. We see them more frequently than specialists, unless we have a condition that requires specialized attention, and even if we have consulted with a specialist, we're usually referred to the GP for routine follow-up. The GP is trained in general medicine and can give advice on general areas of health concerns. Some are accredited in a subspecialty, such as counseling.

Most GPs just want to take care of their patients without the complications of added expenses of technology and long-distance medicine. Nonetheless, it is inevitable that electronic links will become less expensive, allowing GPs more affordable access to the technology required for their offices.

Some GPs will resist change and will continue to interact with their patients in the traditional face-to-face manner. Likewise, many patients will resist the changes that come with the decreased "hands-on" aspect of the physical interaction from the doctor.

As telemedicine becomes more sophisticated, GPs will likely work more closely with health-care institutions and specialists. As a result, more people living in rural, remote areas or those needing home care will benefit. Many people will benefit from being able to have consultations at home using interactive devices that will be as inexpensive and available as TV sets.

As you become more aware of the capability of virtual/telemedicine, you might also choose a doctor who uses this new technology. You might increase your consultations with virtual-docs as well as with your GP. Then again, you might want to continue communicating with your doctor as you do now.

In the future you might have even more options to choose from. The way you communicate will also broaden and change. It will be your choice to keep abreast of new approaches and language needed to achieve optimum communication with your doctor.

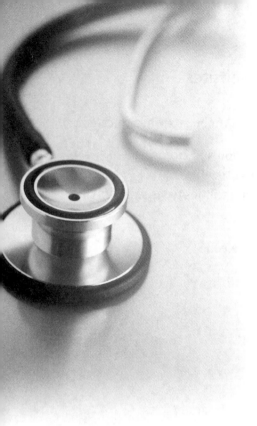

Resources

The following include American and Canadian resources.

1. United States

American Medical Association (AMA): Code of Medical Ethics

http://www.ama-assn.org/ama/pub/physician-resources/medical-ethics/code-medical-ethics.page

1.1 Medical associations

American Medical Association (AMA)

www.ama.ca

American Public Health Association (APHA)

www.apha.org/

Royal College of Physicians and Surgeons of America

www.rcpsus.com

1.2 Other informative US websites

Ambulatory Health Care
http://www.faqs.org/health/topics/31/Ambulatory-health-care.html

Division of Health Facilities Evaluation and Licensing
(State of New Jersey Department of Health)
http://www.state.nj.us/health/healthfacilities/types.shtml#TOP

Eligibility with Medicare
http://www2.eligibilitywithmedicare.com/

Mayo Clinic
www.mayoclinic.org

National Patient Safety Foundation
http://www.npsf.org/

Obamacare Facts
http://obamacarefacts.com/whatis-obamacare/

US Department of Health & Human Services
http://www.hhs.gov/healthcare/rights/law/

White House Health Reform
http://www.whitehouse.gov/healthreform

2. Canada

Canadian Medical Association (CMA): Code of Ethics
http://policybase.cma.ca/dbtw-wpd/PolicyPDF/PD04-06.pdf

2.1 Medical associations

Royal College of Physicians and Surgeons
http://www.royalcollege.ca

The College of Family Physicians of Canada
www.cfpc.ca

2.2 Other informative Canadian websites

Canadian Healthcare Network
http://www.canadianhealthcarenetwork.ca/

Canadian Institute for Health Information (CIHI)
http://www.cihi.ca

Health Canada
http://www.hc-sc.gc.ca/index-eng.php

Regulatory transparency and openness
http://www.hc-sc.gc.ca/home-accueil/rto-tor/index-eng.php

Patients Canada
http://www.patientscanada.ca/

Public Health Agency of Canada
http://www.phac-aspc.gc.ca/

The Top 10 Walk-in Clinics in Toronto
http://www.blogto.com/city/2013/11/the_top_10_walk-in_
clinics_in_toronto/

3. Disease-Specific Websites

amfAR (AIDS foundation, United States)
http://www.amfar.org/

Aids Society (Canada)
http://www.cdnaids.ca/

Alzheimer's Association (United States)
http://www.alz.org/

Alzheimer Society
http://www.alzheimer.ca

Arthritis Foundation (United States)
http://www.arthritis.org/

Arthritis Society (Canada)
http://www.arthritis.ca/

Breast Cancer Foundation (United States)
http://www.abcf.org/

Breast Cancer Foundation (Canada)
http://www.cbcf.org

Cancer Society (United States)
http://www.cancer.org/

Cancer Society (Canada)
http://www.cancer.ca

Diabetes Association (United States)
http://www.diabetes.org/

Diabetes Association (Canada)
http://www.diabetes.ca/

Heart Association (United States)
http://www.heart.org/HEARTORG/

Heart & Stroke Foundation (Canada)
http://www.heartandstroke.com

National Institute of Mental Health (United States)
http://www.nimh.nih.gov

Mental Health Association (Canada)
http://www.cmha.ca/

Multiple Sclerosis Association of America (MSAA)
http://www.mymsaa.org/

Multiple Sclerosis Society of Canada
https://beta.mssociety.ca/

North American Menopause Society (United States and Canada)
http://www.menopause.org/

Center to Advance Palliative Care (CAPC) (United States)
http://www.capc.org

Hospice Palliative Care Association (Canada)
http://www.chpca.net/

Schizophrenia and Related Disorders Alliance of America (SARDAA)
http://www.sardaa.org/

Schizophrenia Society of Canada
http://www.schizophrenia.ca/

4. Internet Support Groups

American Family Care
www.americanfamilycare.com

Doctor on Demand
www.doctorondemand.com

HealthCentral
www.healthscout.com

HealthTalk
http://www.healthtalk.org

5. Virtual Medical and Telemedicine Websites

Canadian Virtual Hospice
http://www.virtualhospice.ca/

HealthCare International
http://www.healthcareinternational.com

Institute for Safe Medication Practices Canada
http://www.ismp-canada.org

Mobi Health News

http://mobihealthnews.com

Virtual Health Group

http://virtualhealthgroup.com/

6. Additional Reading

6.1 Books

Adler, Ronald B., and Russell F. Proctor II, 2013. Looking Out, Looking In (14th edition), Cengage Learning.

Beebe, Steven A.; Susan J. Beebe; Mark V. Redmond, 2013. Interpersonal Communication: Relating to Others (7th edition), Pearson.

Cohen-Cole, Steven A., 2013. The Medical Interview: The Three Function Approach (3rd edition), Saunders.

Fisher, Roger, and William L. Ury, 2011. Getting to Yes: Negotiating Agreement without Giving In (Revised edition), Penguin Books.

Hekmat-panah, Javad, MD, 2013. Communication with & on Behalf of Patients: Essentials for Informed Doctor-Patient Decision Making (1st edition), CreateSpace Independent Publishing Platform.

Lutz, William, 1997. The New Doublespeak: Why No One Knows What Anyone's Saying Anymore (1st edition), Perennial.

Meichenbaum, Donald, Dennis, C. Turk, 1987. Facilitating Treatment Adherence: A Practitioners Guidebook (1st edition), Springer.

Wood, Julia T., 2012. Interpersonal Communication: Everyday Encounters (7th edition), Cengage Learning.

6.2 Self-Counsel Press Eldercare Series

Butler, Lynne, 2008. Protect Your Elderly Parents: Become Your Parents' Guardian or Trustee (1st edition), Self-Counsel Press.

Howe, Tanya Lee, 2013. Supporting Parents with Alzheimer's: Your Parents Took Care of You, Now How Do You Take Care of Them? (1st edition), Self-Counsel Press.

Lauber, Rick, 2014. Caregiver's Guide for Canadians (2nd edition), Self-Counsel Press.

6.3 Websites

"Communicating with Your Doctor," National Coalition for Cancer Survivorship, 2014.

http://www.canceradvocacy.org/resources/communicating-with-your-doctor/

"Communicating with Your Doctor," UCSF Medical Center, 2014.

http://www.ucsfhealth.org/education/communicating_with_your_doctor/

"Effective Patient Communication," Trisha Torrey, 2014.

http://patients.about.com/od/therightdoctorforyou/a/docpatient-comm.htm

"Talking to Your Doctor," National Institutes of Health (NIH), 2014.

http://www.nih.gov/clearcommunication/talktoyourdoctor.htm

"Vanessa's Law Honours Memory of Tory MP Terence Young's Late Daughter," HuffPost, 2013.

http://www.huffingtonpost.ca/2013/12/06/vanessas-law-terence-young-tory_n_4399937.html

"What Is Palliative Care?" Mount Sinai Hospital, 2014

http://www.tlcpc.org/palliative-care

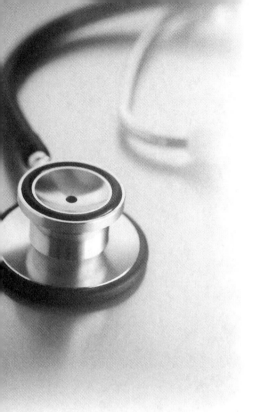

Download Kit

Please enter the URL you see in the box below into your computer web browser to access and download the kit.

www.self-counsel.com/updates/talkdoc/15kit.htm

The download kit includes:

- Checklists
- American and Canadian resources